Diabetes Management Services: A Pharmacist's Resource Guide

Diabetes Management Services: A Pharmacist's Resource Guide

APhA

American Pharmacists Association
Washington, D.C.

Managing Editor: Vicki Meade, Meade Communications
Acquiring Editor: Sandra J. Cannon
Copy Editor: Paula Novash
Editorial Assistant: Kellie Burton
Proofreader: Amy Morgante
Indexer: Suzanne Peake
Layout and Graphics: Michele A. Danoff, Graphics by Design

Published by the American Pharmacists Association
2215 Constitution Avenue, N.W.
Washington, DC 20037-2985
www.aphanet.org

APhA was founded in 1852 as the American Pharmaceutical Association.

To comment on this book via e-mail, send your message to the publisher at aphabooks@aphanet.org

Library of Congress Cataloging-in-Publication Data

Diabetes management services : a pharmacist's resource guide / American Pharmacists Association.
p. ; cm.
Includes bibliographical references and index.
ISBN 1-58212-062-5
1. Diabetes—Programmed instruction. 2. Diabetes—Examinations, questions, etc. 3. Pharmacists—Programmed instruction.
[DNLM: 1. Diabetes Mellitus—drug therapy. 2. Community Pharmacy Services—organization & administration. 3. Pharmacists. WK 815 D53565 2004] I. American Pharmacists Association.

RC660.D4518 2004
616.4'62'0076—dc22

2003028157

How to Order This Book
Online: www.pharmacist.com
By phone: 800-878-0729
VISA®, MasterCard®, and American Express® cards accepted

Contents

Lists OF FORMS AND SAMPLE DOCUMENTS

Appendix A: Forms

Appendix B: Sample Documents

Foreword

Every 24 hours in the United States:[1]

- 75 people lose their eyesight from diabetes.
- 180 amputations are performed because of diabetes.
- 120 people begin treatment for end-stage kidney disease.
- 575 people die from diabetes and its complications.

In 1990, only four states reported a prevalence of diabetes greater than 6%. In contrast, by 2010 more than 10% of all Americans will have diabetes.[2] Currently 18.2 million Americans—6.3% of the population—are thought to have diabetes, now regarded as the sixth leading cause of death in this country.[1]

Women and minorities are disproportionately affected. About 9% of all women have diabetes, but roughly a third of them are undiagnosed. The prevalence of diabetes is two to four times higher among women who are African American, Hispanic, Native American, and Asian/Pacific Islander.

Diabetes creates serious problems in the next generation. As many as 10% of babies born to women with diabetes who receive no preconception care have major congenital malformations.[3] In addition to the staggering human costs of pain, suffering, disability, and death, the economic costs of diabetes are astronomical as well. In 2002, $1 of every $5 spent on health care was for diabetes.[4] The National Committee for Quality Assurance (NCQA) notes that hospital costs for improper preventive care related to control of glycosylated hemoglobin alone is $138,000,000 per year.[5]

NCQA states that 57,000 people die each year because they do not receive appropriate health care, and that 50,000 of those deaths are from known conditions that are not adequately monitored or controlled. A key problem is the health care system's delay in adopting technology and disseminating information to patients and providers that can improve outcomes. Furthermore, NCQA says physicians and other health care providers use evidence-based medicine inconsistently, organizations fail to collaborate to address local health care issues, and existing health care financing provides few or no incentives for excellence.[5]

According to the Centers for Disease Control and Prevention, our current health care system does not do a good job of meeting the needs of people with diabetes despite increases in our knowledge of the disease and treatment options.[6]

These are sobering facts. Can anything be done? In a recent article, pharmacy professor and diabetes expert Stuart Haines notes that implementing a team approach to care improves diabetes management.[6] Increasingly, pharmacists are members of these teams, providing such services as education, screening, and medication monitoring as they work collaboratively with physician colleagues to help patients meet their goals.[7]

The Asheville Project illustrates the impact of pharmacists' services in improving diabetes patient outcomes and reducing costs. In a partnership with local pharmacists, the City of Asheville decreased its health care costs between $1,600 and $3,300 per patient over 5 years, cut sick days in half, and brought the average glycosylated hemoglobin reading to 6.8%.The strong philosophic and financial commitment of the City of Asheville enabled local pharmacists to rearrange their workflow and staffing patterns to offer effective, appropriate services. As a result, medication adherence and persistence increased, and patients were treated with more aggressive regimens and for previously unrecognized or untreated conditions.[8]

Thanks to unique training in the use of medicines and accessibility in communities throughout the country, pharmacists are in an ideal position to change the way the people with diabetes receive care. Most state pharmacy and medical practice acts have been amended to recognize expanded roles for pharmacists in collaborative drug therapy management.[9]

The impetus for writing this book is the stark reality of the diabetes epidemic as well as pharmacists' tremendous potential to improve care by working collaboratively with health care providers and patients. We hope this book will give you the tools you need to assume a significant role on the diabetes care team and launch new services for patients.

Given that diabetes-focused pharmacy practice models are evolving daily, we have organized this text into four sections that we believe provide support to the broadest cross-section of practitioners.

The first chapter, Diabetes and the Pharmacist's Role, by Jean-Venable "Kelly" Goode, David Nau, and Cherokee Layson-Wolf, is the culmination of a diabetes-focused community pharmacy residency project. The project included a 2001 survey of pharmacy-based diabetes patient-management services in community and ambulatory care settings and development of a "how to" document. Chapter 1 reports the results of the survey, gives insights into workable strategies, and provides a framework for initiating diabetes-focused patient care services in pharmacy settings.

In Chapter 2, Business Planning Template for a Diabetes Care Practice, David Medvedeff shares a user-friendly way to create a business plan in a format sure to be familiar to any pharmacist—that of a clinical paper. Without proper business and economic planning, even the most well-intentioned program will fail.

After the business plan is put into effect, you need a quality improvement program to keep the service competitive. Because data collection is critical to quality improvement, you also gain a rich source of marketing data to show potential purchasers of the service. In Chapter 3, Building a Quality Improvement Program for Pharmacy-Based Diabetes Services, David Nau and Virginia Scott offer practical tools and techniques.

Chapter 4, Achieving an ADA-Recognized Practice, by Magaly Rodriguez de Bittner, is a step-by-step guide to help pharmacies receive recognition by the American Diabetes Association. As far as we know, this chapter is the only pharmacy-specific guide for this highly beneficial credential. ADA recognition indicates that an education program meets national standards for diabetes self-management education and opens the door to reimbursement by insurers.

Among steps toward insurance reimbursement was the expansion in 1998 of the Medicare Balanced Budget Act of 1997 to include payment for outpatient diabetes self-management training services provided by certified providers and for glucose monitors, test strips, and other monitoring supplies. Under regulations established in 2001, diabetes education programs with ADA recognition—including those based in pharmacies—can apply for a Medicare provider number. This means that ADA-recognized pharmacy providers can be reimbursed for diabetes education services given to eligible Medicare recipients.

Although this text focuses on diabetes, we believe that pharmacists have an obligation to treat the entire patient—which means also addressing diseases that are not diabetes related and resolving any drug-related problems a patient has. The information in this text can be used not only for diabetes services, but also to create a comprehensive pharmaceutical care practice.

Despite the many challenges facing health care—and especially pharmacy—we're optimistic that you can create a patient-focused practice that is professionally satisfying and economically viable. We hope that this text is a meaningful addition to your library and a valuable tool as you make pharmacy-based diabetes management services a reality.

Anne Burns, RPh
Director, Professional Practice Division
American Pharmacists Association

William M. Ellis, RPh, MS
Executive Director/Chief Executive Officer
APhA Foundation
December 2003

References

1. Centers for Disease Control and Prevention. *National diabetes statistics fact sheet: general information and national estimates on diabetes in the United States, 2002.* Atlanta, GA: US Department of Health and Human Services, Centers for Disease Control and Prevention; 2003.

2. Centers for Disease Control and Prevention (CDC). Behavioral Risk Factor Surveillance System. Available at: www.cdc.gov/nccdphp/aag/aag_ddt.htm#1. Accessed December 5, 2003.

3. *Fact Sheet: Women and Diabetes.* Washington, DC: American Diabetes Association; 2002.

4. American Diabetes Association. Economic costs of diabetes in the US in 2002. *Diabetes Care.* 2003;26:917-32.

5. National Committee for Quality Assurance. *State of Health Care Quality 2003.* Washington, DC: National Committee for Quality Assurance; 2003.

6. Haines ST. The diabetes epidemic: can we stop the spread? *Pharmacotherapy* 2003;23(10):1227-31.

7. Centers for Disease Control and Prevention. *Team care: comprehensive lifetime management for diabetes.* Atlanta, GA: US Department of Health and Human Services, Centers for Disease Control and Prevention, National Center for Chronic Disease Prevention and Health Promotion; 2001.

8. Cranor CW, Bunting BA, Christiansen DB. The Asheville project: long-term clinical and economic outcomes of a community pharmacy-based diabetes care program. *J Am Pharm Assoc.* 2003;43:173-84.

9. American College of Clinical Pharmacy, Hammond RW, Schwartz AH, et al. Collaborative drug therapy management by pharmacists. *Pharmacotherapy.* 2003;23(9):1210-25.

Acknowledgments

Interestingly, this book never started out to be a book at all. What existed almost 2 years ago was a series of diabetes-related initiatives. However, a book evolved because of our sincere interest in helping people with diabetes receive pharmaceutical care services and because of the collaborative spirit among American Pharmacists Association members, elected leadership, and staff of both APhA and the APhA Foundation.

We would like to thank the many dedicated people who made this book possible:

- **The APhA Foundation's Advanced Practice Institute classes of 2001 and 2002.** These cutting-edge practitioners identified the information they needed to grow their practices and, as such, helped create the outline for many sections of this book. Their input was invaluable as the authors drafted and refined their chapters.

- **Tom Stewart, a community pharmacy resident who diligently helped to conduct the survey of pharmacist-provided diabetes patient management services.** His work is sincerely appreciated, as is the participation of pharmacists who gave their valuable time to complete the in-depth phone interview required for the survey.

- **Contributing authors David Nau, Ginger Scott, David Medvedeff, Jean-Venable "Kelly" Goode, Magaly Rodriguez de Bittner, and Cherokee Layson-Wolf.** Their outstanding efforts made this resource a reality. Originally, some of these individuals were asked to develop a monograph and some were asked to develop a lecture with a handout. However, because of their high degree of professionalism and their willingness to contribute their talent and energy for the benefit of others we now have a valuable text. These authors also waived their right to book royalties so that a portion of the proceeds could support the work of the APhA Foundation. We sincerely thank them for their generosity and salute them for their tireless pursuit of excellence.

- **David Nau for his expertise and time in editing this book.** David was instrumental in reviewing and integrating all the pieces, and his efforts as the volunteer editor are sincerely appreciated.

- **Aventis Pharmaceuticals for supporting the Diabetes-focused Community Pharmacy Residency Project.** This project led to the creation of Chapter 1, Diabetes and the Pharmacist's Role.

- **APhA Foundation staff members Dan Garrett and Cindy Wicht.** Their behind-the-scenes efforts helped make this book concept a reality and keep the project on track. Their vision and teamwork allows the Advanced Practice Institute to be an annual forum that generates new thinking and supports practitioners in enhancing their diabetes care services.

Anne L. Burns
William M. Ellis

Contributors

Magaly Rodriguez de Bittner, PharmD, BCPS, CDE
Associate Professor
University of Maryland School of Pharmacy
Baltimore, Maryland

Jean-Venable Goode, PharmD, BCPS
Associate Professor
Virginia Commonwealth University School of Pharmacy
Richmond, Virginia

Cherokee Layson-Wolf, PharmD
Assistant Professor
University of Maryland School of Pharmacy
Baltimore, Maryland

David Medvedeff, PharmD, MBA
Clinical Coordinator
Provider Synergies
Trinity, Florida

David P. Nau, PhD
Assistant Professor
Center for Medication Use, Policy and Economics
University of Michigan College of Pharmacy
Ann Arbor, Michigan

Virginia Scott, PhD
Associate Professor
Department of Pharmaceutical Systems & Policy
West Virginia University School of Pharmacy
Morgantown, West Virginia

Chapter 1

DIABETES AND THE PHARMACIST'S ROLE

Jean-Venable Goode, David Nau, and Cherokee Layson-Wolf

IN THIS CHAPTER:

- Pharmacists' Impact on Diabetes Care Outcomes
- Basics of Diabetes Education and Management
- Training and Credentials
- Recognition for Diabetes Self-Management Programs
- Diabetes Patient Management Services (DPMS) Survey Results
- Strategies for Developing Diabetes Patient Management Services

The Impact of Diabetes

The Centers for Disease Control and Prevention (CDC) has reported that the prevalence of diabetes rose dramatically during the 1990s.[1,2] In 1990, approximately 4.9% of Americans had been diagnosed with diabetes, while an estimated 7.3% of Americans had diabetes in 2000. Nearly 800,000 new cases of diabetes are diagnosed each year, of which 90% to 95% are Type 2 diabetes. Even more people than that have undiagnosed diabetes or impaired glucose tolerance. Coupled with dramatic increases in obesity, the epidemic of diabetes is likely to escalate in the coming decade.

The long-term costs of uncontrolled diabetes are very high. People with diabetes incur health care costs that may be four times as high those incurred by the general population.[3] Cumulatively, people with diabetes accounted for approximately $98 billion in health care expenditures in 1997. Many of these costs are associated with managing the complications of diabetes, such as myocardial infarction or ischemic stroke, which have been estimated to cost $27,630 and $40,616, respectively.[4,5] Health plan costs for patients with diabetes who develop end-stage renal disease typically exceed $53,000 per year.

However, the American Diabetes Association (ADA) estimates that the complications and costs of diabetes could be reduced dramatically if patients maintained adequate control of their diabetes. Results from the Diabetes Control and Complications Trial (DCCT) suggest that intensive treatment and monitoring for persons with Type 1 diabetes could reduce the risk of retinopathy (76%), nephropathy (50%), neuropathy (60%), dyslipidemia (34%), and cardiovascular disease (41%).[6] Additionally, the United Kingdom Prospective Diabetes Study (UKPDS) found that intensive glycemic control of persons with Type 2 diabetes can reduce the overall rate of microvascular complications by approximately 25%.[7] When better glycemic control is achieved, the costs of diabetes decrease significantly.[8,9,10]

In recent years, many health plans have begun to implement disease management or case management programs for their members with diabetes. Several studies have shown that disease management services are effective at improving the quality of care for persons with diabetes, which often translates into monetary savings for the health plan.[11,12,13] These programs often rely heavily on nonphysician providers of care to facilitate patient education, more intensive patient monitoring, and better communication between providers, caregivers, and patients. Because of the importance of medications in the control of diabetes, as well as the frequent interaction of pharmacist and patient, pharmacists have an excellent opportunity to positively impact their patients with diabetes. The goal of this publication is to offer insight to community/ambulatory-based pharmacists on developing diabetes patient management services (DPMS) and demonstrating their value to patients and payers.

Pharmacists' Impact on Diabetes Care Outcomes

Since 1995, there have been numerous studies of the impact of pharmacists' care on the health of persons with diabetes. A variety of outcomes have been assessed including clinical parameters (e.g., blood glucose, low-density lipoprotein cholesterol, hemoglobin A1c, blood pressure), humanistic concerns (health-related quality of life, satisfaction), and costs/expenditures for care. A description of these studies follows.

In 1995, Van Veldhuizen-Scott and colleagues reported their assessment of a pharmaceutical care model for patients with diabetes.[14] They added a pharmacist intervention (either group education or individualized education/monitoring) to an existing multidisciplinary diabetes education program. The patients receiving individualized monitoring were contacted twice monthly for 2 months. At the end of 2 months, the patients who received the pharmacist intervention demonstrated greater knowledge of diabetes medication management and a more positive perception of the pharmacist. Additionally, the patients in the pharmaceutical care model experienced a greater reduction in average blood glucose values as compared to the patients who received only the standard diabetes education program.

During 1997, Fincham and Lofholm collected data from 10 community pharmacists regarding 51 patients with diabetes who were enrolled in a pharmacist-care program.[15] The patients were assessed at baseline and after 2 months in the program. The average hemoglobin A1c of the study patients decreased from 10.6% to 8.7% during the study. Self-reported adherence to the diabetes care regimen also improved, as did the patients' satisfaction with the pharmacy. Health-related quality of life improved in seven of eight domains of the HSQ-12, a questionnaire that measures health-related quality of life. Fincham and Lofholm also found that expenditures on prescription and over-the-counter products increased significantly over the 2-month study, and the number of days of missed work decreased. The pharmacists estimated the number of physician, hospital, and emergency center visits avoided as a result of their care. Using standard estimates for the costs of these visits, the investigators projected that the pharmacists' care resulted in an average cost-avoidance per patient of $4,295.

Coast-Senior and colleagues examined the impact of diabetes care rendered by pharmacists in a Veterans Affairs Health Care System (VAHCS) clinic in Pittsburgh.[16] Patients with difficult to control Type 2 diabetes were referred to the clinic by their primary care providers. The pharmacists provided diabetes education, medication counseling, monitoring, and insulin initiation/adjustments. Twenty-three veterans were followed for an average of 27 weeks. During the study period, the patients experienced significant improvements in hemoglobin A1c and fasting blood glucose concentrations. The average A1c changed from 11.1% at baseline to 8.9% at the final assessment, while the average fasting blood glucose concentration fell from 219 mg/dL to 154 mg/dL.

Pharmacists in a VAHCS clinic in California also demonstrated the positive impact of pharmacists on veterans with diabetes. Gong, Hasson, and Lum studied 81 veterans who were assigned to either a traditional primary care model for diabetes or a diabetes disease management clinic (DDMC) in which a pharmacist or nurse practitioner provided education, monitoring, and dosage adjustments under protocol.[17] Patients who received care in the DDMC experienced a significant improvement in glycemic control. The median hemoglobin A1c fell from 11.4% at baseline to 9.8% at follow-up, while patients in the primary care model did not achieve significant reductions in A1c.

Pharmacists in Asheville, North Carolina, implemented a diabetes care program for self-insured employers in 1997.[18-19] On average, patients experienced a significant reduction in hemoglobin A1c during their first 12 months in the program. This reduction persisted for many patients over a 5-year period. The majority of patients also experienced a reduction in low-density lipoprotein (LDL) cholesterol. Patients' satisfaction with pharmacy services improved significantly and health-related quality of life did not deteriorate during the first year of enrollment. Furthermore, the payers experienced a decrease in total direct medical costs. Employees of the City of Asheville who participated in the diabetes care program decreased their utilization of sick days, which led to greater productivity. The city valued its increase in productivity at $18,000.

Berringer and colleagues reported the outcomes of a diabetes monitoring program at two community pharmacies in Virginia.[20] This program was integrated with the dispensing system in that data were collected from patients at the time of each medication refill. Patients were instructed on the use of blood glucose meters and they provided monitoring results to the pharmacists at each visit. Patient charts were reviewed at a later time when pharmacists were free of dispensing responsibilities, and the pharmacists provided recommendations to the patient's physician when necessary. Over the course of a year, 23 patients who participated in the program and regularly monitored their blood glucose experienced significant improvements in glycemic control. The average fasting blood glucose values for this group changed from 179 mg/dL at baseline to 148 mg/dL at 12 months.

The impact of New Jersey pharmacists on diabetes outcomes was reported by Baran and colleagues.[21] Ten community pharmacists provided diabetes education to 88 patients via 1-hour sessions held every other month for 6 months. Patients were asked to provide copies of laboratory reports and blood pressure readings. For the 20 patients who shared their hemoglobin A1c results, there was a significant improvement in glycemic control. Improvements were also seen in blood pressure and total cholesterol. The number of self-reported physician visits and hospital admissions decreased while the self-rated general health of patients improved over the 6-month period.

Irons and collaborators at Texas Tech University conducted a study of diabetes care provided in a physician-supervised, pharmacist-managed primary care clinic.[22] They compared the glycemic control of 87 men with diabetes whose drug therapy was managed by a pharmacist to a control group of 85 similar patients whose care was not augmented by a pharmacist. The patients in the pharmacist-managed clinic were more likely to achieve an A1c level below 7% when compared to the control group (relative risk = 5.19, confidence intervals = 2.62 to 10.26). The frequency of hypoglycemic events did not differ between the groups. The average number of unscheduled clinic visits related to diabetes was higher in the control group, however. Thus, the pharmacist-managed patients were more likely to achieve optimal glycemic control and less likely to need unscheduled visits.

The positive impact of pharmacists has also been demonstrated in minority populations. For example, Davidson, Karlan, and Hair implemented a pharmacist-managed diabetes care program in a free medical clinic that served a poor, minority population.[23] The pharmacist provided diabetes care according to physician-designed algorithms including the initiation/adjustment of therapy, ordering of laboratory tests, and limited physical assessment of patients. Patients in an experimental group (n = 79) received the pharmacist-care program while a control group (n = 73) received standard medical care at the clinic. The patients in the pharmacist-care group experienced a significant reduction in A1c while the control group showed no improvement. Patients with proteinuria were more likely to be treated with an ACE inhibitor if they were in the pharmacist-care group.

Jaber and colleagues also demonstrated the positive impact of pharmacists working in a clinic that served an urban, minority population.[24] Clinic patients with Type 2 diabetes were randomly assigned to either a pharmacist-based care program (intervention group) or standard medical care (control group). Patients in the intervention group received instruction from the pharmacist on diabetes management including lifestyle modification, medications, and blood glucose monitoring. The pharmacists also ordered laboratory results, monitored patients' adherence to the lifestyle changes and drug therapy, and adjusted the medication regimen as necessary. Patients returned to the clinic every 2-4 weeks for 4 months. Over 4 months, the 17 patients in the pharmacist-care group experienced a significant improvement in glycemic control. The average A1c for these patients changed from 11.5% at baseline to 9.2% at the final visit. The control group exhibited no change in A1c.

Several recent studies have examined the impact of the pharmacist on managed care enrollees with diabetes. Gerber, Liu, and McCombs compared the health care costs of Kaiser-Permanente members with diabetes who visited either an enhanced-care pharmacy or a traditional pharmacy.[25] The patients who visited the enhanced-care pharmacies were presumed to have received additional counseling and monitoring. The estimated total expenditures for patients who patronized the enhanced-care pharmacies were significantly less than the expenditures of patients in the traditional model.

Kelly and Rodgers evaluated the impact of pharmacist-managed diabetes services on several clinical outcomes for patients in a managed care group in Virginia.[26] Patients were referred to the pharmacist-based service by their physicians. They received self-management training, dosage adjustments, and periodic assessments of treatment goals by the pharmacists. When compared to historical controls, the patients who participated in this service experienced a significant improvement in glycemic control. The average A1c of patients in the pharmacist-based service declined from 9% at baseline to 7.5% at the end of 7 months. There was no significant change in LDL or blood pressure for the participating patients.

Nau, Blevins, and Neal showed that community pharmacists could perform ongoing monitoring of key clinical outcomes to identify managed care enrollees with diabetes who were not reaching therapeutic goals.[27] Pharmacists in the Ohio Valley Pharmacist Care Network (OVPCN) performed assessments of hemoglobin A1c, lipids, blood pressure, weight, diabetes knowledge, and medication adherence for patients who visited their pharmacies and who were enrolled in a particular health maintenance organization (HMO). The pharmacists' baseline assessments found that the following percentages of their patients with diabetes were not achieving the therapeutic goal for a particular measure: A1c (63.9%), LDL (69.8%), blood pressure (58.3%), and body-mass index (61.9%). By sharing the patients' clinical data with their physicians, the pharmacists and physicians were able to collaboratively identify problems and revise the patients' therapeutic regimens. The cumulative data were also helpful to the managed care organization for quality improvement.

In a follow-up to the aforementioned study, Nau and Ponte evaluated whether the OVPCN pharmacists' diabetes care program was successful at improving clinical outcomes.[28] The pharmacists provided an individualized education program (three 1-hour sessions) for each patient in addition to quarterly follow-up visits to assess the patient's progress. For 32 patients who completed an average of 9 months in the OVPCN program, the average A1c of the group dropped only a small amount. However, 22 of the 32 patients began the program with a baseline A1c below 8% (indicating reasonable control). For the 10 patients who entered the OVPCN program with a baseline A1c greater than 8%, the average A1c declined significantly from 9.8% to 8.6%. Additionally, the average total cholesterol and LDL decreased significantly across the entire 32 patients. This led the authors to conclude that pharmacist-care programs may be useful for all patients with diabetes, regardless of baseline glycemic control.

In summary, it appears that pharmacists working in community/ambulatory care settings can implement diabetes patient-management programs that positively impact patients and lower the total costs of care. Many of the pharmacist-based programs demonstrated the ability to achieve significant reductions in A1c and some also demonstrated improvements in LDL. Several studies also estimated that the cost savings achieved through reductions in hospital visits far outweigh the typical compensation to pharmacists for diabetes management.

The Pharmacist's Role in Caring for Patients with Diabetes

Pharmacists in all practice settings are in a key position to start providing care to people who have diabetes or are at risk of developing it, or to expand and improve their care. Pharmacy programs for patients with diabetes involve activities ranging from identifying and referring at-risk patients, to supporting ADA-recognized multidisciplinary diabetes care programs. Several areas exist for pharmacists to be involved in caring for patients with diabetes. These are listed in the box below.

Opportunities for Pharmacists to Care for Patients with Diabetes

Some ways in which pharmacists can get involved in caring for patients who have or are at risk for developing diabetes include:

- Identifying patients at risk for Type II diabetes due to known risk factors:[29]
  - — Obese (BMI ≥ 25 kg/m²)
  - — Age over 45 years
  - — Family history of diabetes, especially first-degree relative
  - — Hypertensive (≥ 140/90)
  - — HDL ≤ 35 mg/dL and/or triglyceride level ≤ 250 mg/dL
  - — Diagnosis of gestational diabetes mellitus (GDM) or giving birth to babies over 9 pounds
  - — Member of a high-risk ethnic population (African American, Asian American, Hispanic, Native American, and Pacific Islander)
  - — Impaired glucose tolerance or impaired fasting glucose on previous testing
- Conducting blood glucose screening of patients with risk factors
- Offering point-of-dispensing services including reminders for proper preventive care and glucose testing
- Disease state management
- Providing patient education (including multidisciplinary programs)

Pharmacists should evaluate their knowledge and skills related to diabetes prior to implementing a service for patients with diabetes. A later section will cover available training programs and credentialing. The following box lists the core competencies of a pharmacist providing care to patients with diabetes.

Core Competencies for Pharmacists Providing Diabetes Care

1. Identify the risk factors for diabetes and appropriately triage patients at risk.
2. Discuss and follow the ADA Standards of Medical Care for Patients with Diabetes Mellitus.[28]
3. Assess and educate patients on the following topics:
   A. Consequences of poor glycemic control.
   B. Relationship between diet, exercise, and pharmacologic therapies including lifestyle changes.
   C. Pharmacotherapy of insulin and oral agents including role, proper use, and management of adverse effects.
   D. Symptoms, treatment, and prevention of hypoglycemic and hyperglycemic reactions.
   E. Care of skin, feet, and eyes, oral hygiene, and immunizations.
   F. Treatment of cuts, scratches, and infections.
   G. Proper identification, such as wallet cards and jewelry.
   H. Monitoring parameters including blood glucose testing, ketone testing, and hemoglobin A1c interpretation and record keeping.
   I. Acute and chronic complications.
   J. Comorbid disease states and the related lifestyle changes and pharmacotherapy that are necessary.
   K. Prescription and nonprescription drugs for patients with diabetes.
4. Identify local and national resources for people with diabetes.
5. Describe insurance coverage for supplies and cognitive services.

Basics of Diabetes Education and Management

KEYS TO GOOD GLYCEMIC CONTROL

The ADA has developed the *Standards of Medical Care for Patients with Diabetes Mellitus*,[30] which include specific recommendations for health care providers and for patients with diabetes. Specific goals of treatment are addressed for patients with Type 1 and Type 2 diabetes including complications such as retinopathy, hypertension, nephropathy, cardiovascular disease, and dyslipidemia. Guidelines are provided for health care providers for initial visits and continuing care. Adherence to the *Standards of Medical Care* should lead to better patient outcomes. Therefore, health care providers who use the *Standards* for assessing patient status are better able to improve the outcomes of their patients with diabetes.

STANDARDS FOR DIABETES EDUCATION

The ADA has also established the *National Standards for Diabetes Self-Management Education*.[31] These *National Standards* offer guidance for structure, process, and outcomes for a diabetes self-management education (DSME) program. The ADA created an education recognition program to identify programs that provided high-quality diabetes education as evidenced by adherence to the *National Standards*. Any program interested in receiving recognition from the ADA must follow the *National Standards*, although the curriculum for the education program may be developed using one of two recommended curricula: *Life with Diabetes: A Series of Teaching Outcomes* by the Michigan Diabetes Research and Training Center, or *A Core Curriculum for Diabetes Education* from the American Association of Diabetes Educators (AADE). The *Life with Diabetes* series may be purchased from the ADA website at www.diabetes.org and the *Core Curriculum* may be purchased from the AADE website at www.aadenet.org.

There is an application process through which the ADA assesses whether a diabetes education program meets the *National Standards*. The 6th edition application for ADA recognition is available on the ADA Web site at www.diabetes.org/professional/recognition/erp.jsp. In order to achieve ADA recognition, pharmacy-based programs must have the characteristics listed in the box on the following page.

Features Required for ADA Recognition of Pharmacy-Based Programs

1. **A Certified Diabetes Educator (CDE).** The educator may be a pharmacist.
2. **Advisory team.** The program must maintain a multidisciplinary advisory team that oversees planning.
3. **Data on the population.** The program must collect 6 months of data on the patient population receiving the diabetes self-management education.
4. **Multidisciplinary team.** The team must include a nurse and dietitian. The program must keep a record of all instructors and their credentials, including the continuing education (CE) they have earned. Instructors must have completed 3 contact hours in diabetes specific topics, 3 contact hours in behavioral and learning topics, and 1.5 contact hours in diabetes-related topics in the prior 12 months.
5. **Curriculum.** The curriculum must have measurable learning objectives.
6. **Education records.** The pharmacy program must have permanent records that include the individual needs assessment; medical, diabetes, and social history; education plan; interventions; evaluation of progress; and means of collaboration between team members.
7. **Continuous quality improvement.** The program must have documentation of a continuous quality improvement process to evaluate the effectiveness of the diabetes self-management education.
8. **Behavioral outcomes.** The program must identify and track participant behavioral outcomes (e.g., the proportion of patients who adhere to their self-monitoring plan).

Several pharmacies have been successful in obtaining ADA recognition for their DSME. Tips on how to obtain recognition for your program are addressed in Chapter 4.

TRAINING

Most pharmacists seek additional knowledge and training before providing disease state management services. The type of training may range from learning how to set up services to spending time with an expert in the specific disease state. National pharmacy associations offer certificate programs for pharmacists in developing pharmaceutical care programs and improving their skills in taking care of patients with chronic conditions. Some manufacturers also offer specific training programs for health care providers. For example, LifeScan offers a continuing education (CE) certificate program for pharmacists that consists of intensive self-study and a 3-day live finishing course. Several universities also offer CE and certificate programs for disease state management, some examples of which appear in Table 1-1.

It is important to know that these programs offer a certificate of completion and not board certification. Even after completing a certificate program, pharmacists must engage in lifelong learning about the specific disease state. Among ways to keep up to date on advancements in care of patients with diabetes are attending local, state, and national meetings (including meetings or workshops by the ADA or AADE), subscribing to journals or Web-based information sources, and networking with other pharmacists who provide diabetes services.

CREDENTIALING

Pharmacists can receive diabetes-related credentials in one of three ways:

1. Becoming a Certified Diabetes Educator (CDE).
2. Earning board certification in advanced diabetes management.
3. Receiving credentials in diabetes disease state management.

All three of these credentials are discussed in more detail below. The CDE is especially useful because the ADA will not recognize a diabetes program unless one of its health care providers is a CDE.

Certified Diabetes Educator

The AADE has published both the *Scope of Practice for Diabetes Educators* and the *Standards of Practice for Diabetes Educators*.[32] The AADE defines a diabetes educator as a health care professional who has mastered the core

TABLE 1-1. Examples of Certificate Training Programs

Organization	Program	Web Site/E-mail
American Pharmacists Association	Pharmaceutical Care for Patients with Diabetes	www.aphanet.org/education/ctp/diabetespat.html education@aphanet.org
National Community Pharmacists Association	Diabetes Care	www.ncpanet.org/nipco/diabetes.shtm info@ncpanet.org
LifeScan	Pharmacy Partners in Diabetes Care	www.lifescan.com/professionals/ppdc.html
University of Tennessee	Diabetes Patient Care Certificate Program	http://cop.utmem.edu/pharmacy/CE/default.htm gfarr@utk.edu

of knowledge and skills in the biological and social sciences as well as in communication, counseling, and education, and who has experience in the care of people with diabetes. Since 1986, the National Certification Board for Diabetes Educators (NCBDE) has offered certification in the field of diabetes education. The purpose of the certification process is to provide a mechanism for recognizing clinicians who have met rigorous education and experience requirements in the area of diabetes education. The process for obtaining CDE credentials includes the steps outlined in the box to the right.

Steps for Obtaining CDE Credentials

1. Meet eligibility requirements:
   A. Hold an active, unrestricted pharmacy license in the United States.
   B. Have a minimum of 2 years of professional practice experience in diabetes self-management education in the United States.
   C. Have a minimum of 1000 hours of diabetes self-management education experience within the past 5 years.
   D. Maintain current employment in a primary role as a diabetes educator for a minimum of 4 hours per week.
   E. Submit a completed, current Application for Certification Examination for Diabetes Educators and pay the required fee by the application deadline.
2. Pass the Certification Examination for Diabetes Educators.
3. Maintain certification.

For More Information on the Certification Examination for Diabetes Educators

The National Certification Board for Diabetes Educators (www.ncbde.org) has information on exam content, fees, and renewal of certification. Also, an exam application and handbook may be obtained from:

Applied Measurement Professionals, Inc.
ATTN: NCBDE Coordinator
8310 Nieman Road
Lenexa, KS 66214
Phone: (913) 541-0400
Fax: (913) 541-0156
E-mail: info@goamp.com

Board Certification in Advanced Diabetes Management

In 2001, a new credential was created by the AADE, the American Dietetic Association, and the American Pharmacists Association (APhA) to recognize individuals with advanced knowledge in managing patients with diabetes as well as skills in research, publications, mentoring, and continuing professional development. The process for obtaining Board Certification-Advanced Diabetes Management (BC-ADM) includes the steps outlined in the box below.

One of the main differences between the BC-ADM and the CDE is that even though the credential is available to different disciplines, the BC-ADM test is specific to each discipline. Currently, the ADA does not recognize the BC-ADM for diabetes self-management programs, but discussions are under way for changing this.

Process for Obtaining BC-ADM

1. Meet eligibility requirements:
   A. **License.** Be an active unrestricted licensed pharmacist.
   B. **Education.** Have an advanced degree (masters or doctorate in pharmacy) or currently practice in a state-recognized collaborative diabetes clinical practice.
   C. **Experience.** Have at least 800 hours of clinical diabetes experience within 48 months prior to application.
2. Pass the examination. Information about the exam can be found at www.aadenet.org/ProfessionalEd/credentialing.html.

The domains of the test are:

- Clinical practice (majority of exam)
- Health promotion/health education
- Collaboration
- Research
- Leadership and professional practice

3. Maintain certification by earning 150 hours of CE every 5 years or by being retested.

NISPC Credential in Diabetes Disease State Management

The National Institute for Standards in Pharmacist Credentialing (NISPC) was established by APhA, the National Association of Boards of Pharmacy (NABP), the National Association of Chain Drug Stores (NACDS), and the National Community Pharmacists Association (NCPA) to provide a consistent and objective credentialing mechanism for providers of disease state management. The credentials are awarded to pharmacists who achieve passing scores on disease-specific examinations developed by NABP for NISPC. The DSM examinations are standardized assessment tools developed by a coalition of recognized experts drawn from all areas of pharmacy practice to measure the knowledge and judgment of the pharmacist. The examinations are designed for pharmacists with 2 or more years of practice experience, but any pharmacist with an active license in good standing issued by a board of pharmacy in a U.S. jurisdiction is eligible to participate. As this book goes to press, the price for the first examination is $250. Additional information about the DSM examination is available at www.nabp.net or www.nispcnet.org

The examination includes general competencies in the area of pharmaceutical care as well as specific standards and objectives for each disease state.[33] Specific objectives for the diabetes DSM examination are listed in the box below.

Objectives for the Diabetes DSM Exam Through NISPC

1. Patient Data Collection
   A. Conduct patient interviews pertinent to diabetes.
   B. Compile medical history.
   C. Obtain accurate and relevant physical assessment and laboratory information.
   D. Collaborate with patient's health care providers to secure pertinent information.
2. Patient Assessment
   A. Review and interpret data.
   B. Evaluate current therapy.
   C. Develop a problem list.
3. Patient Care Plan
   A. Develop a pharmacist care plan including therapeutic goals, recommendations for therapy, education needs, and follow-up.
4. Patient Care Evaluation
   A. Assess established parameters at appropriate intervals.
   B. Assess the safety and effectiveness of the patient's therapy.
   C. Assess patient compliance or medication misuse.
   D. Assess adverse reactions, interactions, and/or contraindications.
   E. Assess alternative therapies and interventions in situations where the desired outcome is not being achieved.
5. Documentation
   A. Record and maintain data essential to the continuity of care consistent with applicable laws, regulations, and standards of practice.
   B. Transfer information consistent with federal and state laws

OBTAINING ADA RECOGNITION FOR DIABETES SELF-MANAGEMENT PROGRAMS

The primary reason for pharmacies to obtain ADA recognition for a diabetes self-management program is because it is one criterion for receiving Medicare compensation for DSME. However, other benefits include enhanced marketing of the program by using the ADA education logo, free publicity on the ADA Web site, and referrals from local ADA offices. ADA recognition status is awarded for up to 3 years. In-depth information about seeking ADA recognition can be found in Chapter 4.

Possible barriers to pharmacies achieving recognition include not having access to other members of the health care team (dietitians and nurses), lack of space for group education, and lack of certification. Collaboration is the key to overcoming the multidisciplinary team barrier. Pharmacy representatives should assess current relationships in order to build the diabetes team. If a relationship exists with a physician, assess whether any of the nurses or dietitians in the practice are interested in providing diabetes education. There may be dietitians in private practice in the community who are interested in partnering in a diabetes program.

Often it is not economically feasible to hire a full-time dietitian or nurse, but offering a fee for time spent with patients is realistic. If space is not available for group education, the pharmacy could still offer individual education. Pharmacists should document time spent with patients in diabetes self-management education because documented patient-care time is required when you apply for CDE credentials or for ADA recognition of your program.

A Profile of Diabetes Patient Management Services (DPMS)

In developing this resource manual, a survey was conducted of pharmacists who have implemented diabetes services in the community, either based in community pharmacies or in ambulatory care settings (clinics or physicians' offices). The purpose of this survey was to characterize the various DPMS already in place and to identify the key strategies that lead to the successful establishment of DPMS.

SURVEY METHODS

Pharmacy-based DPMS sites were identified across the country through various means: e-mail soliciting participants, word of mouth, and referrals from current practitioners or academicians. Pharmacists at the identified sites were initially contacted by letter, then by telephone, to solicit their participation in the survey. If the pharmacists were interested in participating, a 30-45 minute phone interview was scheduled for a later date. An interviewer then called the participating pharmacists at the agreed-upon time and conducted a structured interview. The interviewers for this project were two community pharmacy residents (one each from West Virginia University and Virginia Commonwealth University). Of 75 programs identified, interviews were completed with 30. The most common reason given for nonparticipation was lack of time. All interviews were completed by March 2001.

Participants were asked questions in several categories: site characteristics, program design, implementation strategies, and compensation for services. Additionally, the pharmacists were asked to share any "words of wisdom" that they thought would be helpful to other pharmacists who seek to create similar services. The responses were transcribed and analyzed by the project team (Goode, Nau, Layson-Wolf, Stewart).

RESULTS

Site Characteristics

Participating Sites

See Figure 1-1 for the various types of participating sites. A majority (17) of the sites were independent community pharmacies.

Prescription Volume

Nearly all (27 of 30) participants reported average daily prescription volumes of less than 400 per day. Figure 1-2 presents the distribution of prescription volumes for the participants. The five sites that reported zero prescription volume were predominantly ambulatory care clinics. The prescription volume was similar across all other categories of participants (independent, chain, supermarket).

Figure 1-1.
Participating Sites

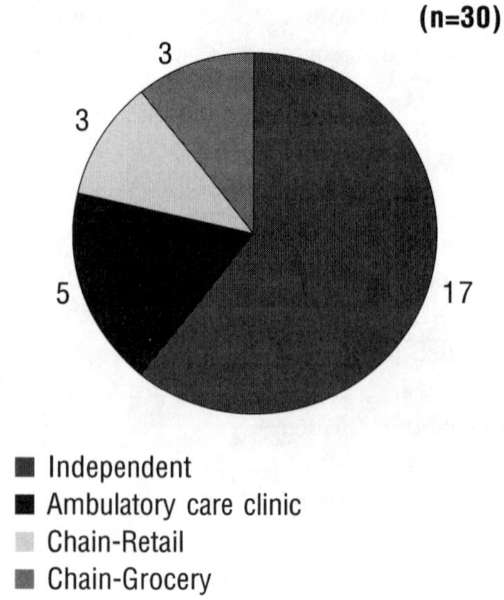

Figure 1-2.
Average Daily Prescription Volume

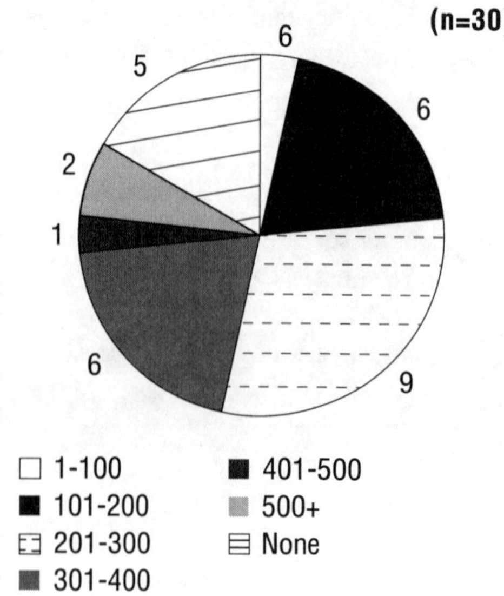

Academic Affiliations

A majority of the programs had some relationship with a college or school of pharmacy. Eleven programs served as clerkship sites for pharmacy students, and 11 sites had pharmacists who were adjunct faculty. Twelve of the sites had pharmacists who serve as assistant or associate professors. Thirteen programs also had community pharmacy residents. Such relationships can be of extreme benefit to programs because they can help provide up-to-date information resources and care practices. They can also assist in grant funding and by promoting networking and exchange of ideas with other programs.

Longevity of DPMS

A surprising finding was that eight programs were initiated 5-10 years ago, with two programs having been initiated more than 15 years ago. Twenty programs were initiated within the past 5 years, four of which were initiated within the past year. This provides evidence that pharmacists have long identified the need for diabetes programs within the community.

Structure of DPMS

Facilities

Sixteen of the 30 sites had either a semi-private area or a private consultation room/office where patient care is provided. Thirteen of the sites used a combination of semi-private/private consultation area, conference-style room, and/or off-site facilities. One program conducted its activities off-site only. Twelve sites had preexisting facilities when implementing their DPMS, although not all had been built specifically for patient care programs. Six sites redesigned the entire pharmacy, while another six added a new counseling area. Five sites incorporated a combination of structural changes, which also included a reconfiguration of workflow to accommodate the program.

External Resources

During program planning, it is necessary to consult various resources. The distribution of resources used can be found in Figure 1-3. Manufacturers appeared to be a large resource for program development, with professional associations such as APhA, NCPA, and the ADA also being consulted. Surprisingly, very few programs consulted other pharmacists (7) or other programs (1) that were currently involved in DPMS.

Staff Utilization

Most sites reported that two pharmacists were providing diabetes care. However, the pharmacy staff involved in a DPMS need not be limited to pharmacists. Technicians (12) and/or billing clerks (7) played roles in a majority of the surveyed programs. They assisted with patient recruitment, billing for blood glucose meters, and scheduling patient appointments. Programs are also incorporating staff not normally found in the community pharmacy: dietitians (4) and nurses (1). This is of importance because these two professionals are required members of ADA-recognized programs. Pharmacy residents (13) and students (11) have also been identified as members of the DPMS team.

Figure 1-3.
Resources Used in Program Development

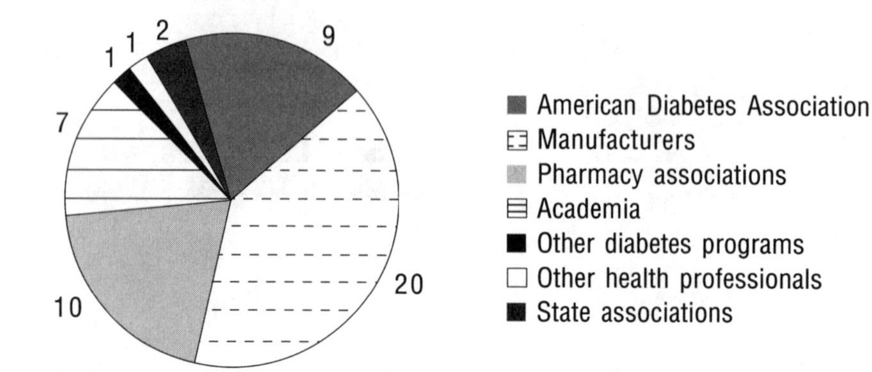

Training/Recognition

Most sites reported participation in formal training programs in preparation for the DPMS. Certificate programs (APhA, NCPA, the National Institute for Pharmacist Care Outcomes, state associations) were used most (15). Nine sites also reported receiving training from either manufacturer programs (4) or university-based programs (5). Pharmacists in four programs reported having previous pharmacy residency training. All sites required some sort of training for participating pharmacists from either formal or informal training programs, continuing education, or certificate programs.

At the time of the survey, only one program interviewed had achieved ADA recognition. There was one CDE involved in this program. Four programs were in the process of applying for recognition. Of the four programs applying for recognition, all had pharmacists with CDEs actively participating in the program. [Editor's note: By October 2003 there were at least 25 ADA-recognized diabetes education sites based in community pharmacies.]

DPMS Components

Diabetes management programs may contain several different components: individual counseling, group education sessions, patient monitoring, and drug-therapy management. Most sites (19) provide only individual counseling, while only one program is conducting solely group education. The remaining programs are using a combination of the two basic educational structures.

The depth of educational services provided can depend on the desired scope of the DPMS. Disease and dietary education were provided by all the programs. Twenty-six of the 30 programs also provided blood glucose monitor training, with fewer sites reporting insulin-injection training (2) or physical activity instruction (3).

Patient monitoring services reported by the participants included: laboratory values (22), drug therapy monitoring (20), and foot exams (12). While nearly all sites monitored blood glucose and/or A1c, many sites also monitored blood pressure and lipid levels. In some cases, the test was conducted in the pharmacy while in other cases, the pharmacist obtained the laboratory results from the laboratory or physician's office.

Documentation

Nineteen of the programs surveyed used hard copy charts for patients and completed either preprinted forms (17) or used free-form documentation (2). Twelve programs reported using some sort of computer-based charting system. Free-text charting can be created with word processing software or can be kept within the patient record on the pharmacy's prescription record system. Other sites used one of the following computer programs created specifically to track patient data: Tiara, CarePoint, Diatrends, Informacare, Softcare. Some sites also used software provided by blood glucose meter manufacturers to download information on blood glucose trends.

Scheduling

Eighteen of the sites scheduled appointments with patients, while nine allowed for either appointments or walk-ins. The remainder provided services on a walk-in basis only. The timing of the scheduled appointments varied greatly by site. Some scheduled appointments before or after normal business hours, while some chose "slower" times of the day or shift overlap times.

Patient Recruitment, Program Promotion, Participation

Recruitment methods can vary depending on resources and the patient population. Word of mouth—or point of sale—promotion is perhaps the simplest and most inexpensive means to recruit patients. Fourteen programs reported using this method; 20 programs, however, reported receiving patients through physician referrals. Eighteen programs reported detailing the DPMS directly to physicians and other health care providers, while only one program directly promoted the DPMS to employer groups. Nine programs also reported receiving referrals from nurses, two from dietitians, and two from case managers. Five programs reported receiving referrals from other pharmacists.

None of the programs used one single method of promotion and recruitment. In addition to point of sale promotion, many programs participated in health fairs to generate awareness of the DPMS and a few also used newspaper, radio, or Internet advertisements.

Programs were asked to report the number of patients participating at the time of the interview. The patient load of the programs varied greatly, from having very few patients (< 10) to a large number of patients (> 200.) Programs with larger groups of patients were the ambulatory care clinics interviewed. Figure 1-4 shows the number of patients enrolled in DPMS. Although eight sites had only 1-10 patients each, six sites had more than 100 patients each.

Figure 1-4.
Number of Patients Enrolled in DPMS

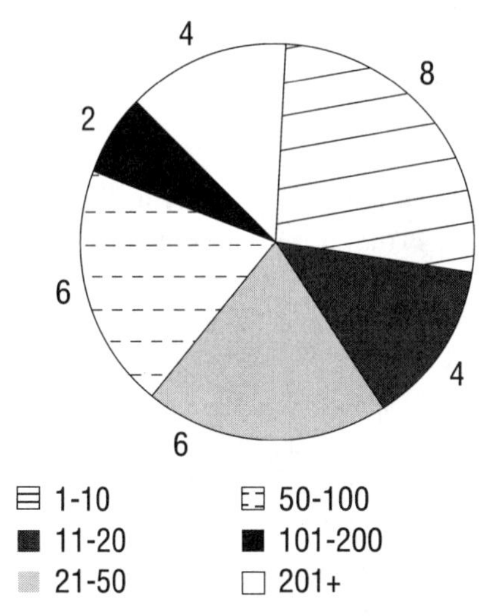

Compensation

Obtaining compensation for services is a constant struggle for pharmacists. Most programs interviewed (14) used a combination of out-of-pocket and third-party billing to obtain compensation for services rendered in their DPMS. Only two programs reported providing services at no charge as a value-added service. Nine programs obtain only out-of-pocket compensation, three programs charge only third parties for services, and two programs obtain compensation through physicians billing third parties for services. Figure 1-5 shows programs' compensation types.

Figure 1-5.
Compensation Type

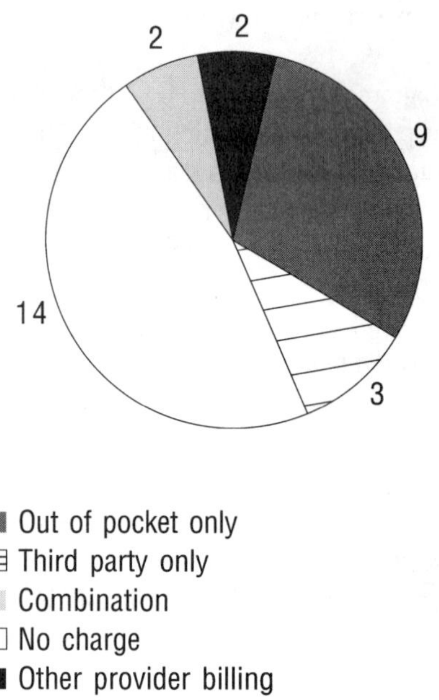

Documentation of Clinical Impact

Fifteen of the participating sites had documented the clinical impact of their program in a structured manner. The most frequent criteria used to establish the impact of the program were changes in glycemic control (as measured by hemoglobin A1c, blood glucose, and number of hypoglycemic episodes), as well as lipid and blood pressure control. Six of these sites have reported their impact via publications, abstracts, or presentations.

Barriers

The programs reported several barriers to providing care. Lack of perceived need by patients and physicians was the most frequently reported barrier (13), with compensation for services (9), cost of program implementation (8), and physician resistance (7) being the others reported the most.

Words of Wisdom from Survey Participants

At the end of the interview process, programs were asked for their "words of wisdom" for those interested in establishing a DPMS. Here is a small sampling of their suggestions.

- **"Strategy, strategy, strategy."**
—The development of a program must be approached systematically. Use the planning tool recommended earlier to assist in program planning.

- **"Opportunities are endless, marketing is key."**
—Lack of perceived need by both patients and health care providers is a barrier that most programs will encounter. Due to the high incidence of diabetes in the community, there is an endless need for such programs. Develop a good marketing plan to educate the public about your program and its benefits.

- **"Use your resources well, learn from what others have done."**
—Do not feel you need to reinvent the wheel. Several persons, such as those interviewed for this paper, have taken their own steps to create a program. Networking is an excellent way to create your own individualized program. These programs can share what has worked and what has not worked. Creating a connection between your program and others can also create a support system for all programs involved.

- **"Persistence. Initially, your expectations may be large, but in the end, it really happens in little steps. Do it little by little."**
—Successful programs take a long time to create. A stepwise process is necessary to create a realistic, working program. Paying attention to detail will benefit the program in the long run. Persistence and motivation are very strong keys to creating and maintaining a successful DPMS.

- **"Learn to think outside the box."**
—Creativity is an important aspect of making your program unique. There may be programs in existence already in your community. You will need to determine how you can distinguish your program from others by adding a unique benefit to your list of services.

APPLICATION OF SURVEY RESULTS

The interviews conducted for the survey provide very important information regarding the current status of DPMS around the country. All programs demonstrated similarity in educational and management concepts, but at the same time each exhibited unique characteristics. The information in the previous section provides examples to assist you in developing your programs. The next section discusses our recommendations on the steps that should be taken to develop your own DPMS.

Strategies for Developing Diabetes Patient Management Services

To develop an effective, successful DPMS, careful planning must take place. Using a stepwise process to guide the development of the DPMS helps identify various needs, obstacles and barriers, goals and objectives, and other aspects important to program planning. The steps described in the following section provide a framework for creating your own DPMS. Formalized implementation plans, or business plans—vital aspects of creating successful patient care programs—are discussed as well. Additional information on business plans is available in Chapter 2.

Steps in Planning and Developing Your DPMS

Step 1. Do Foundational Planning
- A. Conduct a needs assessment
- B. Evaluate your ability to meet needs
- C. Identify barriers
- D. Prepare a mission statement
- E. Develop program goals and objectives
- F. Determine services to provide
- G. Plan a timeline to implementation

Step 2. Delineate Program Specifics
- A. Structure of program
- B. Staffing, time, and space issues
- C. Documentation systems
- D. Equipment and lab requirements

Step 3. Determine Compensation Systems
- A. Identify different routes of compensation
- B. Determine methods for direct billing of third parties
- C. Decide how much pharmacists get paid for a DPMS
- D. Assess whether compensation will exceed costs
- E. Determine how to develop a compensation system

Step 4. Determine promotion/advertising strategies

Step 5. Evaluate quality and costs for continual improvement

STEP 1: DO FOUNDATIONAL PLANNING

A. Conduct a Needs Assessment

Before implementing any patient care service, it is usually best to assess the needs of your patients and of other health care providers or insurers in your geographic area. Diabetes is a widespread disease, affecting people of many age groups, and it is very likely that DPMS programs would be helpful in any practice. However, it will still be useful to characterize the diabetes population in your area.

A simple approach for evaluating the patients at your practice site is to analyze prescription records (e.g., run an audit trail on prescriptions for diabetes medications and products). Determine the number of patients with diabetes at your site and how many are using insulin versus oral agents. Then take into account the population characteristics of your practice site (ethnic and age demographics, urban versus suburban, income level, cash-paying versus third-party insured, etc.). Characterizing your target population will help you determine the optimal type and level of services.

The easiest way to determine the needs or desires of your patients is to talk to them about diabetes services, either informally with individual patients or in a formal focus group. For example, you could find out if they have ever participated in a diabetes education class or met with a dietitian. Has anyone explained why and how to monitor their blood glucose? Asking about the problems they encounter or their concerns and questions should give you a better idea of what patients want. Often, patients have many questions but are reluctant to ask. They think we are too busy, or they don't want to appear ignorant or "whiny." It's best to set up a time to meet with the patients or ask that they write down concerns. Avoid hitting them "cold" with your inquiry when they are hurriedly picking up a prescription.

It's also useful to meet with local physicians, dietitians, and diabetes educators. You need not meet with all providers, but should target those who are influential, who send many patients to you, or with whom you have built an established relationship. Such meetings can help build your professional image by letting other providers know that you are truly interested in helping patients achieve optimal outcomes and that you want to work collaboratively to make the other providers' jobs easier (and yours too).

The majority of pharmacists interviewed in our survey indicated that meeting with providers was one of the most important steps in developing a successful DPMS. If physicians refer patients to you for diabetes management—or even just glucose meter instruction—patients are likely to feel more comfortable about enrolling in your program. A physician's referral may also be necessary to garner compensation from some payers. Collaborative efforts tend to facilitate better communication between you and the physician because you determine together how you want to exchange information and make changes in the patient's therapy.

B. Evaluate Your Ability to Meet Needs

It is important to examine whether you are able to fit the unmet needs you identify. Do this by completing a simple SWOT analysis: S = Strengths, W = Weaknesses, O = Opportunities, T = Threats. See Figure 1-6 for an example of a SWOT chart.

Figure 1-6.
SWOT Analysis Chart

Your Practice Site	
Strengths	Weakness
Outside Forces	
Opportunities	Threats

There are several areas of consideration when completing a SWOT analysis. When considering your practice site, analyze the following:

- **Training.** Has your staff received any training in diabetes education and management?
- **Existing programs.** Does your pharmacy already have existing disease-state management programs that may provide you with a framework to design a DPMS?
- **Other pharmacy services.** Do you offer services that set your pharmacy apart from others in the area?
- **Staff.** Does your pharmacy have adequate staff (pharmacists, technicians, clerks) to support a DPMS?
- **Space.** Does your pharmacy have adequate space to provide patient care services (semiprivate or private counseling area, office, conference room)?
- **Licenses and waivers.** Does your pharmacy have a CLIA (Clinical Laboratory Improvement Amendments) waiver to provide point of care testing? Does your state allow pharmacies to obtain a CLIA waiver? Does your state require licenses for any of the "nonpharmacy" services you intend to provide?
- **Financial status.** Does your pharmacy have funds for developing and supporting a DPMS, increasing pharmacy staff, purchasing equipment, and making renovations to the pharmacy?
- **Workflow.** Does your pharmacy have a good workflow in which technicians are used optimally to allow pharmacists time to provide patient care services?
- **Working relationships with other health care providers.** Does your pharmacy have good working relationships with health care providers who can refer patients to your DPMS? Does your state allow collaborative practice agreements?
- **Patient base.** Does your pharmacy currently have a population of patients who can benefit from a DPMS?

Outside forces can also affect your DPMS. Consider the following areas for opportunities and threats:

- **Health care providers.** Are local health care providers receptive to pharmacy-based patient care services?
- **Third-party payers.** Will third-party payers provide you with a patient base and compensation for services?
- **Patient population.** Is the local patient population receptive to patient care programs, do they see a need for such programs, and are they willing to pay for them?
- **Other diabetes management education groups.** Are there other DPMS providers in the area?
- **Compensation.** Will you be able to obtain compensation either directly from patients or from third-party payers?

A strength of your program, for example, may be that you have a private consultation office at your practice site. An opportunity would be a physician's desire for you to train his or her patients on blood glucose meters. A weakness may be a lack of staffing, and a threat may be a hospital that is offering blood glucose meter training. Conducting a SWOT analysis will help you identify the areas you need to address and develop strategies to overcome potential problems. The challenge is to turn weaknesses into strengths and threats into opportunities.

Once you have answered the above questions, arrange them into their proper space within the SWOT grid in Figure 1-6. At this stage it is important to prioritize your responses because you may not be able to address all the weaknesses and threats you identify. Determine which ones are vital to your program, and create strategies to overcome them.

C. Identify Barriers

After conducting the SWOT analysis, you may encounter potential barriers to the program. These barriers can include resistance from other health care providers, lack of perceived need by both patients and health care providers, lack of compensation for services, and cost of program implementation.[32] This section will discuss barriers in relation to community pharmacy, but these same issues may be applicable to ambulatory care practice.

Health Care Provider Resistance

Community and ambulatory care pharmacists have various levels of relationships with numerous health care providers, such as nurses and physicians. You can build on these already established relationships to create partnerships with other health care providers.

Collaborative practice is a hot topic in the pharmacy world. Now that many states allow for collaborative practice agreements between pharmacists and physicians, opportunities abound for partnerships that can greatly impact the delivery of patient care. If your state laws and regulations explicitly permit formal collaborative practice agreements, take advantage of them. The section below discusses how to initiate relationships that can lead to a collaborative practice agreement in a DPMS. Although it is not always necessary to develop such a formal relationship, it will certainly assist in making a greater impact on improved patient outcomes.

Establish Good Rapport with Local Health Care Providers

Establishing a good relationship with health care providers is the first step in developing a DPMS. When you analyze your current relationships with health care providers, your interactions may range from minimal (new prescription calls and refills), moderate (make recommendations regarding proper dose, drug interactions, etc.), to high (making recommendations regarding proper therapy, reporting patient data, etc.). Most pharmacists would rate their interactions in the minimal to moderate range. These relationships must be expanded for your patient care services to be successful.

McDonough and Doucette define a stepwise process in which relationships can be created with other health care providers.[34]

These collaborative working relationships (CWRs) are vital to the development of collaborative practice agreements. Table 1-2 contains the strategies that McDonough and Doucette state are vital to the different stages of developing CWRs.

In the first stage (Stage 0), "Professional Awareness," the relationship consists mainly of phone interactions between the physician and the pharmacist related to new prescriptions, refills, and adverse drug reactions. Stage 1, "Professional Recognition," is where pharmacists increase the physician's recognition of their services and describe the benefits they would provide to both the practice and the patients. In this dynamic process, the pharmacist's open discussion with the physician allows for changes in the pharmacist's patient care program to best fit the needs of the physician's practice. Although the process may be mainly unilateral in the beginning because more communication is coming from you, the relationship with the physician strengthens as you engage in repeated positive exchanges.

TABLE 1-2. Strategies to Create Effective Working Relationships with Physicians

Stage 0: Professional Awareness Initial stage where pharmacists can position themselves to strengthen relationships with physicians
Stage 1: Professional Recognition ■ Communicate with targeted physicians to inform them of your interest in collaborating. ■ Identify pharmacy services that can complement the physician's practice and meet patient's needs. ■ Discuss ideas with physicians to judge their interest. ■ Refine ideas to meet the needs of physicians with whom the potential for establishing a collaborative working relationship exists. ■ Schedule another face-to-face meeting with the goal of starting to build a collaborative working relationship.
Stage 2: Exploration and Trial ■ Make only high-quality and high-priority recommendations to physicians. ■ Get physicians' feedback about recommendations. ■ Document the outcomes of recommendations. ■ Discuss with the physician the best way to communicate recommendations (e.g., telephone call, fax, progress note, or a combination of these).
Stage 3: Professional Relationship Expansion ■ Communicate to referring physicians the patient outcomes that have resulted from pharmacy care interventions. ■ Be consistent in the provision of care to patients. ■ Continue to make high-quality clinical interventions. ■ Have periodic face-to-face meetings with physicians to establish and enhance personal and professional relationships. ■ Identify any conflicts due to pharmacy care interventions and discuss strategies to resolve them.
Stage 4: Commitment to the Collaborative Working Relationship The authors state that the strategies for Stage 4 are the same as Stage 3. What is most important is the continuation of consistent care and the provision of high-quality clinical interventions.
Source: Adapted from McDonough RP, Doucette WR. Developing collaborative working relationships between pharmacists and physicians. *J Am Pharm Assoc.* 2001;41(5):682-92.

In Stage 2, interactions increase and trust is built between the pharmacist and physician regarding recommendations that have been made. A key strategy is to discuss communication means that would be most useful or convenient for all parties involved in the CWR.

Stage 3 and 4 call for continuous communication between the pharmacist and physician, high-quality interventions, consistent provision of care, and continuous revision of the CWR to identify conflicts and develop a plan to address them.

Nurses are also important to consider when developing CWRs. Some nurses view these types of services as a threat because they are often the ones who have provided patient education within a physician's practice. Talking to some nurses to ascertain the level of education and disease management that they provide to patients with diabetes can help you identify areas of unmet need. When nurses are made aware of the benefits of your services, they may become important referral sources for patients into your program.[35]

Develop Collaborative Practice Agreements

Collaborative practice agreements are an important step in formalizing the relationship between pharmacists, physicians and patients. Currently, 38 states have some sort of statute or regulation governing collaborative drug therapy management. The level of care ranges from educating patients to changing current therapy to having prescriptive authority. Unfortunately, most pharmacists have not taken advantage of the ability to enter into collaborative practice agreements.

First, as discussed above, it's essential to establish a relationship with the physician. Physicians in the following circumstance tend to be easiest to work with:

- Those in a single practice or with one other partner and limited staff.
- Salaried physicians, who are usually required to see a certain number of patients a day. Often they are more than willing to refer more complicated drug therapy patients to pharmacists.

Collaborative practice agreements validate the role of the pharmacist. Having such an agreement in place helps you provide consistent care to patients in your diabetes management service. Although the state governs how the agreement is formalized and the language of the document, you must establish a mechanism for communicating patient progress and complications to the physician. Also, it is a good idea to have regular meetings to discuss patients and philosophy of care.

Lack of Perceived Need by Patients and Health Care Providers

Even if you plan the perfect patient care program, few patients or providers are likely to express interest unless you implement the proper marketing plan. Many patients perceive that their physician and his or her practice will provide all their diabetes education needs. Others may think that they do not need education services. To convince patients of your service's benefits you can offer them "trial" assessments to uncover their educational needs. After obtaining the results you can discuss with them how your program will benefit them and fill their educational needs.

As discussed earlier, other health care providers may feel that they do not need your program's services. Talking with them and providing printed materials about your program—including information on the effects such programs have on patient outcomes—are good strategies for convincing them that you will add to the quality of their patient's care.

Problems with Identification of Resources

In the initial planning stages of DPMS it is vital to identify potential resources, such as information on program development, patient information, and funding. Although a wealth of resources are available, the challenge is knowing where to find them.

Identify Pharmacy Practitioners Who Have Already Developed a DPMS

Why reinvent the wheel? Many pharmacy practitioners have experience developing DPMS and can serve as an information resource for you. Some are not as willing as others to share information, especially proprietary information, but most will offer strategies for developing and implementing a DPMS. Even if no DPMS practitioners are within your geographical location, most are still reachable by phone or e-mail.

Attending pharmacy association meetings can also provide you with a means to network with innovative practitioners. Forums are often held where pharmacists discuss various aspects of patient care services and interact with attendees, allowing you to make connections with people who may assist you. If you view "networking" as a tedious task, keep in mind that it gives you a chance to identify others with common interests and experiences and form supportive relationships.

Many pharmacy associations create networks of practitioners in specialty areas, but sometimes this expertise is left untapped. Openly sharing ideas about innovative practice helps benefit and advance the profession as a whole.

Occasionally pharmacists are reluctant to share information because they fear competition. In reality, however, it is not possible for one practitioner to see all patients—and patients need these important services. Although practitioners may want to protect certain proprietary information, most programs operate on very similar structures. The more pharmacists who provide similar services and the more patients who receive them, the better pharmacists can demonstrate the value of their role and the more firmly entrenched the concept of pharmacy-based diabetes education will become.

Contact Your Nearest Pharmacy School

Many pharmacy schools and colleges have community pharmacy faculty trained in developing and implementing patient care services. They can be a great source of information and assistance. If your pharmacy serves as a clerkship site you may already have good relationships with local pharmacy schools.

Contact Your Local Pharmaceutical Industry Sales Representative

When industry sales representatives call on your pharmacy to detail you about their newest drug products, make the most of your time by asking them how they can support your DPMS. Companies may provide different levels of support, from printed patient education materials (which may or may not contain product-specific labeling) to financial support for your program. Companies that manufacture blood glucose meters provide training in diabetes, such as the "Pharmacist Partners in Diabetes Care" provided by Johnson & Johnson and LifeScan (www.lifescan.com/professionals/ppdc/).

Contact Charitable Foundations or Professional Associations

Local charitable foundations can be an excellent source of startup funds for your DPMS. Although not all foundations focus on the development of health care services, some will consider your proposal if you can establish that the community needs greater services for people with diabetes—especially if you provide some services to indigent citizens. Professional associations or foundations (such as the APhA Foundation or AADE) may also provide starter grants for developing diabetes care programs.

Lack of Pharmaceutical Care Training

A popular definition of pharmaceutical care is: "establishing a therapeutic relationship with the patient, interviewing the patient to collect the data needed to identify drug therapy problems, developing and implementing a patient-specific care plan to resolve the problems identified, providing ongoing monitoring and follow-up services to the patient, and documenting all patient care activities."[36] Some practitioners have not yet embraced this concept.

Although pharmaceutical care is not yet standard practice in traditional community pharmacies, it is vital to the success of a DPMS. Organizations such as APhA provide programs that train pharmacists about pharmaceutical care concepts. APhA, NCPA, and NIPCO provide certificate programs in diabetes and other disease states in accordance with the pharmaceutical care model.

Practice-Related Constraints

Your pharmacy may have many internal barriers to implementing DPMS, including lack of time, finances, space, personnel, and management. These barriers, which must be addressed to ensure success, are examined in the following sections.

In terms of finances, large amounts of money are not always necessary. Although a private patient counseling room is ideal, a small, partitioned-off area may provide adequate privacy for patient counseling until funds can be identified for remodeling. In-store and point-of-sale advertising can be as effective as large, costly marketing plans. In lieu of elaborate documentation software, simple spreadsheets or a word processing program may suffice.

D. Prepare a Mission Statement

A mission statement should demonstrate the philosophy and purpose of your practice. For example, "The mission of Jones Pharmacy is to provide patients with services that improve their health." A mission statement specific to your DPMS might be: "The mission of the Jones Pharmacy diabetes care program is to help our patients with diabetes have better health." This mission statement should be clearly articulated to all of the pharmacy staff and displayed at the practice site so patients and employees are fully aware of your practice philosophy.

Although crafting a mission statement may seem trivial, it's a key reminder to you and your employees that the purpose of your pharmacy is not only to dispense medications, but to provide services that fill patients' needs. Even more important is to back up the "words" with actions that are consistent with the mission.

E. Develop Program Goals and Objectives

Goals and objectives, which enumerate the specifics of your mission statement, must be created early in your program's planning stages. They must establish a clear vision and focus and be achievable.

Goals define what you want to accomplish with your DPMS. Sample goals include:

1. Offer a wide range of diabetes-related products and devices.
2. Provide enhanced medication counseling and glucose meter training to people with diabetes.
3. Conduct assessments of drug therapy via laboratory tests (hemoglobin A1c, lipid profiles), physical assessments (blood pressure, foot exam), and patient interviews.

Objectives establish the specific steps necessary to achieve your goals. They should be realistic and measurable. You should base your objectives on the needs of your target population and prioritize them. For example:

1. One month after completing the education program, 90% of patients will demonstrate adequate knowledge of diabetes and their medications.
2. 100% of patients who were trained to use a blood glucose meter will be contacted 3 months later for reevaluation of meter technique.

The goals and objectives discussed above refer only to DPMS program planning and do not necessarily focus on patient outcomes. As you implement your program and begin to educate and manage patients, patient-based goals and objectives should also be established depending on patients' needs.

F. Determine Services to Provide

Whatever level of services you choose to provide in your DPMS, make sure it is based on the ADA National Standards for Diabetes Self-Management Education Programs.[31] Your level of services should be based on available resources (staffing, space, materials) and the frequency of which services should be provided. Table 1-3 (page 16) lists levels of service and care partners who may participate. Many DPMS programs are initiated with Level 1 services only, which are later built upon. Educating patients about diabetes management is a major focus of most programs (Level 2).

It is easiest to provide Level 1 services because they do not require intensive resources and may already be part of your day-to-day pharmacy practice. However, self-monitored blood glucose (SMBG) and injection training require more skill and involve more time to interact with the patient. Level 2 services involve primary educational services including self-management techniques in foot, skin, mouth, and eye care. Reinforcing these techniques is important to help patients prevent disease complications. If the proper technology is available, downloading SMBG results and explaining them to the patient is also helps reinforce the importance of monitoring blood glucose and examining changes in blood sugar levels.

Level 3 includes services that can enhance or "step-up" the other levels of service, such as providing methods for diabetes patient to interact with each other, share information, and obtain a feeling of support. You can also offer adjunctive clinics in weight loss, smoking cessation, hypertension, or cholesterol monitoring. Level 3 activities, if permitted in your state, provide an excellent opportunity to engage in collaborative practice.

TABLE 1-3. Level of Services to Provide and Possible Collaboration Partners

LEVEL	COLLABORATION PARTNERS
Level 1: Product-Initiated Services	
■ Diabetes medication counseling	Pharmacist
■ Self-monitored blood glucose (SMBG) monitoring	Pharmacist
■ Insulin injection training	Pharmacist, CDE, and Nurse
■ Assistance in selecting nonprescription medications	Pharmacist and Physician
Level 2: Primary Educational Services	
■ Self-management education	Pharmacist, CDE, Dietitian, Nurse
■ Foot care	Podiatrist
■ Skin care	Dermatologist
■ Oral care	Dentist
■ Eye care	Ophthalmologist
■ Downloading/cleaning meters	Pharmacist, Nurse, CDE
■ Blood pressure monitoring	Pharmacist and Nurse
■ Weight monitoring/management	Pharmacist, Nurse, Physicians, Dietitian
Level 3: Services to Add Depth/Breadth to Practice	
■ Diabetes support group	CDE, Pharmacist, Nurse
■ Assistance in adjusting therapy or management tools to improve glycemic control	Pharmacist and Physician
■ Smoking cessation clinics	Pharmacist and Physician
■ Exercise clinics	Exercise trainer
■ Weight management clinics	Pharmacist, Physician, Dietitian
■ Assistance in reducing risk factors for complications	CDE, Pharmacist, Physician
■ Lending library to diabetes resources	Pharmacist, CDE, Dietitian
■ Referral network to other health care professionals	Pharmacist, CDE, Nurse, Dietitian
■ Focused education or "curbside consultation" with other health care professionals	Pharmacists and Nurses
■ Community programs	Pharmacists, Nurses, CDEs
■ Diabetes screenings	Pharmacists and Nurses
■ "Brown Bag" medication days	Pharmacists
■ "Meter" days	Pharmacists, Meter manufacturers
■ Blood testing: A1c and lipids	Pharmacists and Nurses

Source: Adapted from American Pharmacists Association. Pharmaceutical care for patients with diabetes: a certificate program for pharmacists. June 2000.

G. Plan a Timeline to Implementation

Like the famous saying "Rome was not built in a day," neither is a DPMS. Because programs take time to develop and implement, it is important to create a planning timeline. Before you begin to enroll patients you need time to address the issues identified in your SWOT analysis, which may take several months.

Divide your timeline into the following components:

- **Planning:** Conduct a SWOT analysis and develop strategies to overcome barriers.
- **Initiation:** Collect patient education materials and other resources, obtain equipment, and set up your patient care area.
- **Patient Recruitment:** Actively identify and recruit participants.
- **Implementation:** Launch your services.
- **Evaluation:** Continually assess your program's effectiveness and address areas of strength and weakness.

STEP 2: DELINEATE PROGRAM SPECIFICS

A. Structure of Program

The structure of your DPMS program can be individualized (one-on-one), group-based, or a combination of the two. The Centers for Medicare and Medicaid Services (CMS) may pay for group-based education programs of up to 20 participants, with time allotted to assess and follow up on each individual's educational needs.

Group-based education allows you to serve a large number of participants at a time while one-on-one sessions allow for needs assessment and reinforcement of learning. Space is always a consideration for group-based education programs. Most pharmacies do not have conference rooms, but you can circumvent this problem by using rooms in community centers or schools.

B. Staffing, Time, and Space Issues

Staffing is critical. Who will be involved in the program? Pharmacists usually run it and provide most of the care and services, but some programs also involve other pharmacy staff. Pharmacy residents and students, for example, can help with development and implementation; pharmacy technicians can recruit patients and handle dispensing tasks to free pharmacists' time; and billing clerks can ease the process of obtaining compensation for services. Some DPMS programs also have dietitians or nutritionists on staff.

You must decide whether time should be formally set aside for DPMS or whether to provide services on an as-needed basis. If you set aside a few hours a day or a specific day a week, you will need additional staffing during these time to provide adequate coverage in the pharmacy. Some programs hire pharmacists specifically to run the DPMS, and some use residents to provide additional DPMS help. Table 1-4 spells out specific advantages and disadvantages of providing services by appointment during allotted hours or on a walk-in basis.

Whether to schedule DPMS appointments also depends on the extent of services provided and the size of your patient base. If a patient is required to fast before laboratory work, for example, he or she may need an early morning appointment.

Time is of the essence in community pharmacy, and pharmacists' schedules are often filled with dispensing and administrative tasks. We often ask ourselves, "Where does the time go?" McDonough and colleagues suggest carefully evaluating how time is spent in the pharmacy.[35] Such an evaluation is a good way to identify tasks that can easily be delegated to others to free pharmacists for patient care services. The ideal plan is to allocate patient-care time in your daily schedule so it becomes part of the routine.

Staff support is frequently an issue when pharmacists try to find time for patient care services. Hiring new personnel is not always necessary, however. Carefully analyzing staff tasks lets you know which ones can be handled by pharmacy technicians and clerks. Analyzing workflow can help identify what is preventing the timely processing of prescriptions. If you train technicians to handle all dispensing tasks that are nonpharmacist dependent (prescription order entry, counting, packaging medications, etc), you'll have more time to check prescriptions and counsel patients. Your staff can also play key roles in marketing and managing your patient care program, such as passing out flyers to potential patients and scheduling appointments.

In most community pharmacy settings, management support is a must in the development and implementation of DPMS. The management team can provide insight into the finances, staffing, and other resources available for your program, help you with the program's business aspects, and create a supportive atmosphere for your efforts.

TABLE 1-4. Appointments Versus Walk-ins

	ADVANTAGES	DISADVANTAGES
Appointments	■ Able to set aside time for pharmacists and other staff to participate in DPMS activities ■ Allows manager to incorporate the time into staff scheduling and anticipate when extra help will be needed ■ Allows people performing the services to avoid interruptions and rushing through procedures ■ Can be used for both group and one-on-one programs	■ May require extra staffing, including new hires, which may increase the program's budget ■ Requires that appointment times are convenient to patients and not just the pharmacists
Walk-in basis	■ Is most convenient to the patient ■ Reduces the need to set a special schedule ■ May be acceptable for one-on-one programs	■ May be inconvenient for pharmacy staff ■ Delivering proper care may be difficult if there are time constraints ■ Not applicable to group-based programs

Space, of course, is an important consideration. Even if your preexisting pharmacy space does not seem to allow for additional services or your budget for layout alterations is limited, creativity can overcome these obstacles. In most pharmacies, at least a semi-private area can be set up, such as a small table and a few chairs with a portable privacy screen. You can also provide services outside of the pharmacy area—in conference rooms or break rooms—as long as you can maintain patient privacy. You can even provide services in outside facilities, such as community centers, which can help with marketing and visibility.

C. Documentation Systems

Documenting DPMS activities is essential for keeping track of your interactions with patients, especially when multiple pharmacists or technicians need to view their records. Written reports on patients' medication use and objective data such as blood pressure or blood glucose readings help you assess the patients' progress towards therapeutic goals.

A good documentation system will facilitate your quality improvement program, a required element for ADA recognition. The ADA requires that you document patient-related data and periodically review it across your patient population to determine your program's impact and identify areas needing improvement.

Your level of documentation and the forms you use to capture data depend on the services you establish. Often, patient-specific data is recorded on "flow-sheets" or "monitoring forms, examples of which appear in Appendix A at the end of this book.

Preprinted forms are extremely convenient for collecting information and ensuring consistency between patient contacts. Alternatively, a simple method of free-form documentation is the SOAP note (S = subjective, O = objective, A = assessment, P = plan).

Documentation can be kept electronically or in a file cabinet. If you use paper charts, each form should contain the patient's name and be kept in chronological order to prevent confusion.

Some pharmacy-based diabetes programs document interactions in the "notes" section of the pharmacy computer system. These programs, which can be tailored to your needs, allow you to track pertinent labs, goal achievement, and other information.

D. Equipment and Lab Requirements

Using pertinent labs to obtain key measurements (hemoglobin A1c, blood glucose, lipid panels) can help you track patients' diabetes care progress. Although the type of measurement equipment you need depends in part on your breadth of services, it is also regulated by each state under the Clinical Laboratory Improvement Amendments (CLIA). View the CMS website for the latest CLIA updates (www.cms.hhs.gov/clia). Also, CMS and the CDC both set standards for laboratory testing. Requirements for each state can be determined by contacting the state regulatory board that oversees CLIA.

The two levels of CLIA tests are waived testing and moderate complexity testing. The latter has stricter requirements, including a lab director, clinical consultant, and technical consultant. Waived testing does not require these personnel but must still meet certain criteria. To obtain requirements for a "certificate of waiver," contact your local regulatory board. Once obtained, the certificate of waiver must be renewed every 2 years.

Most laboratory equipment used in a DPMS has CLIA-waived status. All members of the pharmacy staff are able to perform CLIA-waived tests provided they have been adequately trained in using the testing equipment (see Table 1-5). An article by Rosenthal gives more detail on how pharmacists can conduct tests via the CLIA waiver process.[37]

Not all states allow CLIA-waived testing in the pharmacy setting. If your state is one of them and you need laboratory results, you can obtain them from the patient's physician. Rapport with the physician can be helpful but it is also important to obtain a release of medical information signed by the patient. Adhering to the confidentiality guidelines of the Health Insurance Portability and Accountability Act is also important.[38]

TABLE 1-5. CLIA-Waived Laboratory Tests

TYPE OF TEST	EXAMPLES
Blood Glucose	
Home Blood Glucose Meters	Accucheck Advantage LifeScan Ultra and OneTouch Profile Precision QID
Blood Glucose and Fructosamine	LXN Duet Glucose Control Monitoring System
Blood Glucose and Ketones	Abbott Laboratories Medisense Precision Xtra, Advanced Diabetes Management System
Cholesterol	ChemTrak Accumeter Johnson & Johnson Advanced Care Cholestech LDX Boehringer Mannheim Accu-Chek Instant Plus Cholesterol Actimed Laboratories, Inc. ENA.C.T. Total Cholesterol Test Lifestream Technologies Cholesterol Monitor Polymer Technology Systems (PTS) MTM Bioscanner 1000 for HDL Cholesterol and for Triglycerides
Fructosamine	LXN Fructosamine Test System LXN IN CHARGE Diabetes Control System
HbA1c	Bayer DCA 2000 Metrika DRx Hb A1c Cholestech GDX
Albumin	Roche Diagnostics Chemstrip Micral
Microalbumin/Creatinine	Bayer Clinitek 50 Urine Chemistry Analyzer
Ketones	PTS Bioscanner for blood ketones

Source: Adapted from Centers for Medicare & Medicaid Services (CMS). Clinical Laboratory Improvement Amendments (CLIA) Program: List of Waived Tests. Available at: http://www.cms.hhs.gov/clia/waivetbl.pdf. Accessed December 1, 2003.

A letter mailed or faxed to the physician that describes your program and is accompanied by a copy of the medical release form will help you obtain the needed lab results. Appendix A at the end of this book contains a sample patient consent for release of medication information (Form 1). It also contains several useful assessment forms (Forms 2-4), as well as a sample letter to the physician (Form 5), screening results form (Form 6), and referral form (Form 7).

STEP 3: DETERMINE COMPENSATION SYSTEMS

Developing compensation systems can be an imposing task for even the most experienced pharmacist. Most pharmacists are very familiar with reimbursement procedures for drug dispensing, but few have billed for patient care services. Fortunately, some pharmacists have been successful at obtaining compensation for their services and can be a model for the rest of the profession.

A. Identify Different Routes of Compensation

Pharmacists have typically billed for their services through one of two routes. Billing through another provider, such as a physician or hospital, was often the only successful way to get compensation when clinical pharmacists first began billing for their consultation services. It is still used by many pharmacists who work as CDEs in hospital-based clinics or physician offices. In this approach, billing for the pharmacist's activities is handled by the staff in the clinic or physician's office who are familiar with billing for professional services.

The second, and increasingly more common route, is to bill the payer—whether the patient or third-party payer—directly. Many patients are willing to pay a modest fee for useful services—although the amount they are willing to pay varies greatly. Some patients cannot afford to pay for all their medications, let alone hundreds of dollars for comprehensive patient-management services. Some patients won't pay for anything, even if they have the funds. Most, however, will pay if they perceive that the potential health benefits of your service outweigh its costs. Thus it's important to help patients understand the benefits and to price services appropriately.

Many pharmacists select a price for "self-pay" patients that is roughly equal to the amount that they would charge a third-party payer. When patients cannot afford the fee and have no insurance that covers the service, some pharmacists provide discount coupons to help them.

Billing directly to third-party payers is the most challenging route for pharmacists. Many payers are still not used to paying pharmacists for anything other than drugs or durable medical equipment (DME). However, some pharmacists have been successful at obtaining compensation directly from Aetna, Prudential, Blue Cross Blue Shield (BCBS), Medicaid, and numerous HMOs.

It is important to understand that many compensation decisions within insurers are made at the local level. Thus, if a pharmacist in Iowa obtains payment from BCBS, it doesn't automatically mean that a pharmacist in Arizona will be paid by BCBS for the same services. Additionally, the amount paid for a particular service will differ among insurers.

B. Determine Methods for Direct Billing of Third Parties

The most frequent mechanism for billing third-party payers is the CMS-1500 form. This form and its companion coding systems for diagnoses (ICD-9-CM) and procedures (CPT) are the standard billing methods all health care providers use. ICD-9-CM stands for International Classification of Diseases, Ninth Revision, Clinical Modification. Current Procedural Terminology (CPT) codes were developed by the American Medical Association and are updated yearly. They are supplemented by CMS's Common Procedure Coding System (HCPCS), used for billing Medicare and Medicaid.

The CMS-1500 form can be sent electronically or printed and mailed to the insurer. In fact, an increasing number of pharmacy computer systems enable the pharmacist to print a completed CMS-1500 form using patient data from the computer and predefined information for common payers.

To complete this form, you will need the diagnosis code for diabetes (generally 250.01 for Type 1 diabetes or 250.02 for Type 2 diabetes, although insurers may accept a generic 250 code) as well as procedure codes. The procedure code for your services will often be negotiated with the payer. Frequently, this may be the CMS code for diabetes education (G0108 for individual sessions or G0109 for group sessions). Sometimes, an evaluation/management (CPT-E/M) code will be used for services other than patient education. The specific CPT-E/M code that you should use depends on whether you are dealing with a new patient or existing patient and on the complexity of the patient visit. Most pharmacists use only a few different codes for their services. Additional details on billing with a CMS-1500 form are available in educational programs from professional associations such as APhA, NCPA, or AADE. Reference materials, such as CPT and ICD-9-CM codebooks, can be obtained from the American Medical Association Press (www.amapress.com).

Some payers require additional information to process payment for a pharmacy-based DPMS, such as a "statement of medical necessity" from the patient's physician. Some pharmacists have prepared preprinted referral forms that physicians can sign for this purpose. These forms can be kept at the physician's office or faxed to the provider when necessary. You may also want to have the patient sign an "assignment of benefits" statement that permits the insurance payment to come directly to you. This statement also indicates that the patient may be responsible for the portion of the fee not paid by the insurer. Patients should also sign a consent form authorizing you to share or receive their medical information with other providers involved in their care.

C. Decide How Much Pharmacists Get Paid for a DPMS

The fee that a third party is willing to pay often depends on the average amount of time or other resources involved in providing the services. Some payers establish fixed fees for a given type of patient encounter and pay only the fixed amount regardless of how much time you spend with a patient. Others allow pharmacists to bill different amounts based on the length of time spent with the patient or the complexity of the patient's health problems. Thus, it is important to find out the payer's policies before you try to submit a bill.

For diabetes education services, many pharmacists have received $75 to $125 per session for individual patient encounters lasting 1 to 1.5 hours each. Sometimes they receive a copayment of $5 to $10 from the patient. Pharmacists who provide only blood glucose meter training frequently report receiving $15 to $30 per session, which typically lasts 15 to 20 minutes. The Medicare reimbursement rate for diabetes education (which is only available to ADA-recognized programs or providers) is $62.74 per hour for individual instruction and $36.73 for group instruction. However, Medicare will only pay for individual instruction in limited circumstances, and it limits the number of education sessions per patient. For the latest rules on Medicare reimbursement for diabetes education, visit www.aadenet.org or http://cms.hhs.gov/medicare.

In addition to diabetes education, pharmacists may also provide diabetes monitoring and management services. Sometimes, this will include conducting a blood pressure assessment as well as tests such as hemoglobin A1c, blood glucose, or cholesterol. Charges for these tests are frequently bundled with education services to simplify payment procedures or because of restrictions within the payer's existing contracts with clinical laboratories. In situations where the payer will compensate the pharmacist for CLIA-waived tests, the Medicare payment rate is usually applied.

D. Assess Whether Compensation Will Exceed Costs

Will the payment you expect to receive for your services exceed their cost? Although it may be reasonable to accept an operating loss on the services in the short run, you must expect some profitability in the future. Keep in mind that the long-term benefits of implementing the service may go beyond revenues directly from the DPMS, such as obtaining new prescriptions or DME business from patients referred to your patient-management services.

The costs of implementing service will vary depending on their scope. Providing enhanced counseling may require relatively little investment if you already have available counseling space. However, setting up pharmacy laboratory services may involve an investment of $5,000 to $10,000. Figure 1-7 describes potential costs to consider when developing a comprehensive DPMS.

E. Determine How to Develop a Compensation System

The most important step in obtaining compensation for patient care services is negotiating with the payer. Some pharmacists have succeeded by sending in a claim form without prior discussion with the payer, but we strongly encourage up-front negotiation with the payer regarding your service and its value.

Figure 1-7.
Estimated Costs for a Pharmacy-Based Diabetes Patient Management Service

Estimated Start-up Costs

Equipment/Supplies:		$ 5,819
DCA 2000 – Bayer Diagnostics	$ 2,500	
A1c cartridges (60)	$ 410	
A1c controls (2 boxes)	$ 170	
LDX Analyzer – Cholestech	$ 1,900	
Lipid profile cartridges (30)	$ 390	
Lipid controls (1 box)	$ 55	
Sphygmomanometer – wall mounted	$ 100	
Scale and counter weight	$ 200	
Sharps container	$ 15	
Lancets (100)	$ 59	
Gloves, swabs, Band-Aids, gauze	$ 20	
Waste Disposal Fee (1 year)		$ 200
CLIA waiver		$ 100
Training (1 pharmacist)		$ 500
Remodeling		$ 500
Advertising/Promotion		$ 500

Assumptions

1. The estimates were based on having sufficient supplies for 30 patients for 1 year.
2. The pharmacy would provide HbA1c, lipid, and blood pressure testing. (A1c 2x/yr; lipids 1x/yr)
3. The "recommended list price" was used for equipment and supplies.
4. The pharmacy would undergo minor physical modifications.
5. The number of staff would not change, nor would overhead (e.g., utilities, rent).
6. Patient education materials were obtained at no cost.

Total Costs: **$ 7,619 ($254/pt)**

At managed care organizations (MCOs), some pharmacists have found an advocate in the director of pharmacy services or director of quality improvement. Many payers, however, do not want to create special contracts or compensation systems for just one pharmacy. They seem more interested in negotiating with a network of pharmacies that can provide a standard benefit throughout the geographic region served by the MCO. Thus, there is strength in numbers.

In all negotiations, be organized and prepared for questions about the structure, benefits, and costs of your services. Some flexibility is also good, but resist the temptation to give away too much just to "get a foot in the door." You need a clear understanding of both the costs involved in your service and the payment that other providers receive for similar services. This allows you to determine whether a competitive price will cover the costs of your investment. Forming a network of diabetes care pharmacies can spread out the costs of implementation (e.g., training, development, or purchase of materials).

One strategy to make your services more financially attractive is to engage in a risk-sharing agreement with the payer. In this approach, the pharmacy and payer share the financial rewards of better care, but also the risk that the services may not lead to cost savings. In other words, if the services reduce the total costs of care for people with diabetes enrolled in a particular health plan, then the pharmacy garners a portion of the savings as payment. If the services do not result in substantial cost savings for the payer, then the pharmacy receives a lower payment for the services. More details on risk-sharing contracts are available in an article by Schwed, Miall, and Harteker.[39]

A current example of applying risk sharing to pharmaceutical care services is the outcomes-based pharmacist reimbursement system developed by Outcomes Pharmaceutical Health Care in Iowa.[40] Within this system, pharmacists are compensated for designated interventions through a payer-funded risk pool. The payers fund the risk pool if the pharmacy providers attain specific performance goals. An intermediary organization processes the pharmacists' claims for interventions and evaluates pharmacist performance.

To begin formulating your compensation system, do the following:

1. Determine who the most common payers are for your patients with diabetes.
2. Investigate whether these patients are currently participating in a diabetes education program.
3. Find out their interest in receiving additional diabetes management assistance from you.
4. Identify other pharmacists in the area who want to collaborate in a diabetes care network.
5. Determine the costs of implementing such a service as well as the typical payments that common payers make for diabetes education.
6. Design your service and determine the price you would like to be paid.
7. Open a dialogue with the payer's director of pharmacy regarding your proposed program.
8. If necessary, ask the pharmacy director to direct you to other key decision makers within the insurer.
9. Describe your services and their value. Be prepared to answer questions about your credentials and your capability to provide services to the insurer's members with diabetes.
10. Consider sharing the risk and be willing to adapt your services to the specific needs of that payer.
11. Be persistent. If the people you speak with are reluctant to move forward with your proposed services, find other advocates such as physicians, patients, or employers. The more "nonpharmacy" voices that speak in favor of your services, the better your chances of reaching agreement.

STEP 4: DETERMINE PROMOTION AND ADVERTISING STRATEGIES

Promotion and advertising are critical to the success of your DPMS. A recent book by Holdford[41] thoroughly reviews the application of marketing principles to pharmacy practice. Here are a few suggestions, however, for promoting a DPMS. You should begin by developing a marketing plan. A good marketing plan begins by defining your product (i.e., the DPMS), the price for your product, and the potential customers or facilitators of your services (i.e., the target audience). The target audience may include patients, caregivers, managed care organizations, employers, pharmacy benefit managers, and other health care providers.

Next, develop goals and strategies for reaching each target audience. One goal may be to make every existing diabetes patient at your pharmacy aware of your DPMS. The strategy for achieving this goal may be to have the pharmacist extend a personal invitation to each diabetes patient when the patient picks up a medication refill.

You may need different promotional strategies depending on your target audience. Examples of strategies include:

- Personal contact
- Brochures
- Letters to patients and physicians
- Press releases
- Announcements
- Newsletters
- Health fairs
- Special events (including open houses for physicians and patients)
- Referral sheets
- Education programs for civic and local diabetes association chapters
- "Shelf talkers"—information about the DPMS placed on the shelf near diabetes products
- Partnerships with industry representatives who already market their diabetes products to health care providers

An "education-based marketing" approach may be particularly useful in promoting your services. In this approach, you provide patients with free educational material about diabetes at the point of dispensing. The material also mentions the availability of diabetes services at your pharmacy and tells the patient how to obtain more information about your services. You can also prepare education-based material for radio, television, or the Internet that helps the public identify you as a diabetes expert.

Your promotional strategies should be evaluated regularly to determine what is and is not working. This will save money and time. Using a variety of strategies may increase the effectiveness of your promotions.

Key Strategies for Success in Your DPMS

Plan

Follow a systematic approach to developing your service. Determine the key service components that will be most highly desired by patients, physicians, and third-party payers in your area to avoid creating a service that won't be used. Early on, identify the costs associated with training, equipment, advertising, and personnel to help you determine the appropriate price and promotional strategy.

Network

Learn from others' successes and mistakes. Attend professional meetings to find pharmacists who have implemented pharmacist care services and struggled with the same issues. Connecting with colleagues who share a common interest will help you identify strategies that have led to success. Their moral support can also keep you moving when you are faced with numerous obstacles and competing priorities.

Maintain Persistence and Creativity

You will inevitably encounter difficulties as you implement your new services. The most successful pharmacists generally find creative ways to overcome these barriers. Rather than giving up when faced with barriers, they persist in their efforts to establish what they perceive as a good service. They tackle one problem at a time and keep moving forward.

A. Use Different Levels of Promotion

Different levels of promotion and advertising can be implemented. The simplest, least costly, and perhaps most effective method is to target the patient at the point of dispensing. Patients with diabetes can easily be identified by their prescription profiles. You can flag these patients' prescriptions so that when they pick up their medication they are invited to talk to the pharmacist.

Pharmacy technicians and clerks can also make patients aware of your diabetes-related services. You can place signs about the program near the diabetic supply aisle and flyers or pamphlets on the pharmacy counter. You can also place flyers at community centers, churches, or offices of physicians, optometrists, and dentists. Obviously, you should obtain permission before posting flyers. Seeking permission to post information about your services may give you a chance to initiate conversations about your services and thus further enhance awareness of the program.

You can send mailings to identified patients, but you must protect a patient's confidentiality when sending items via mail. (For example, do not put any information on an envelope or postcard that identifies the person as having diabetes.) Diabetes screenings are also great ways to target interested patients and provide them with information about the program. Many pharmacists have held a "diabetes day" at the pharmacy to kick off their new services. Patients who use the program are also great resources because they often refer friends and loved ones who may benefit from your services.

More costly methods of promotion include media advertising on television or radio or in newspapers. Creating a Web page for your DPMS can also be helpful. The page could be embedded within your pharmacy's Web site, and could use simple quizzes about diabetes knowledge or information about diabetes to spark people's interest. To help determine the value of promotions and advertising, weigh their expense against the potential increase in use of your diabetes service.

B. Promote to Other Providers

Finally, promote your program to other health care providers. Meeting with them will not only increase awareness of your services, but also help you tailor your services to their needs. Obtaining referrals from health care providers will build a collegial environment, facilitate communication, and allay patient concerns about communication between providers. Although some pharmacists have encountered physicians who are resistant to pharmacy-based DPMS, clarifying your intentions is likely to help minimize confusion or distrust.

When marketing patient care services to physicians and other health care providers, invite them to visit your facilities and see your plans. You could also include the person on an advisory committee, which is a good strategy for obtaining "buy in." Then do your homework so you know how the provider gets paid (salaried, fee for service, capitated, or part of risk-sharing plan). For example, physicians who receive capitated payments may be more willing to refer patients because then they are not losing money for patient care visits of low clinical intensity. Identify the kind of help that the provider desires. Do they want patient education or assistance in selecting cost-effective therapies?

Be Prepared for Physicians' Questions

Always be prepared for a productive dialogue with physicians and other health care providers by knowing the answers to the following questions. Present this information in a clear, concise, polished way.

1. Why do my patients need this service?
2. What is your specific training?
3. What will it cost?
4. Who is going to pay for it?
5. Can you do it? Have you done it?

You want to "get in the back door," which means educating patients, caregivers, and employers about the value of your services and having them inform their providers. It may also be helpful to start by caring for a few patients and use evidence of their positive outcomes as a selling point.

When meeting with physicians to explain your services, it is be best to make an appointment. Appointments early in the day are often best because practice sites become very busy and may fall behind schedule in the afternoon.

Many of the same tips apply when promoting your services to third-party payers. Begin by establishing a relationship with someone in the organization. Volunteer your time to help with committees, such as the pharmacy and therapeutics committee. Offer to participate in educational programs, health fairs, brown bag days, and awareness days or to write an article for their newsletters.

Establishing a relationship with the organization (MCOs, self-insured employers, employers, and pharmacy benefit managers) puts you at the forefront when they begin to think about disease state management programs and compensation. Again, do your homework by learning about the focus of the organization. What are their current efforts? What do they need help with? Review the National Committee on Quality Assurance (NCQA) Health Plan Employer Data and Information Set (HEDIS) requirements to undersand how the organization's performance will be evaluated for accreditation (www.ncqa.org). Be prepared for the same productive dialogue as above and get in the back door using the same strategies.

STEP 5: EVALUATE QUALITY AND COSTS FOR CONTINUAL IMPROVEMENT

Quality improvement is a required component for ADA recognition of your diabetes education program.[31] Adopting the principles of continuous quality improvement (CQI) will help to optimize the performance of your diabetes care program.[42,43] CQI is team-oriented and based on the philosophy that we can always do better. Thus, everyone involved in your diabetes care program should regularly provide input on how the program can be improved.

One of the first steps of CQI is to establish the goals and objectives of your diabetes care program, and prepare detailed plans for implementing the program. You should then determine how you will measure your program's performance and evaluate your progress towards the goals of diabetes management. For example, measurements might include the percentage of patients who score at least 90% on a written test of diabetes knowledge; the percentage who have an A_{1C} of less than 8%; the average satisfaction rating patients give to your program; or the percent of patients who adhere to diet, exercise, or medication regimens. These numerical measures of quality are often called performance indicators. More information on performance indicators and CQI for diabetes management services can be found in Chapter 3.

Your team should meet periodically (e.g., quarterly) to review the latest performance indicator data and discuss how the program might be improved. If changes are warranted, you will be able to track the impact of the changes through subsequent reviews of your performance indicators. Document the minutes of your meetings and keep track of indicator data for ADA recognition.

From a business perspective, it is important to continually evaluate the return on your investment in the DPMS. Pharmacist managers must decide whether the actual revenues from the DPMS warrant continuing the program in its present form. Sometimes modifying price, promotional strategies, or program contents will be necessary to sustain the program.

Organizations Providing Diabetes Resources

EDUCATION AND MANAGEMENT

American Diabetes Association
National Service Center
1701 Beauregard Street
Alexandria, VA 22311
703-549-1500
800-DIABETES
www.diabetes.org

American Association of Diabetes Educators
100 West Monroe, 4th Floor
Chicago, IL 60603
800-338-3633
www.aadenet.org

Juvenile Diabetes Research Foundation
120 Wall Street
New York, NY 10005-4001
800-533-CURE
www.jdrf.org

PROVIDER TRAINING, CERTIFICATION, AND CREDENTIALING

National Certification Board for Diabetes Educators (NCBDE)
330 East Algonquin Road, Suite #4
Arlington Heights, IL 60005
847-228-9795
www.ncbde.org

continued on page 24

Organizations Providing Diabetes Resources, continued

LifeScan Pharmacy Partners in Diabetes Care
LifeScan, Inc.
P.O. Box 504
Newtown, PA 18940
800-227-8862
www.lifescan.com

American Medical Association Press
American Medical Association
515 N. State Street
Chicago, IL 60610
312-464-5000
www.amapress.com

CENTERS FOR MEDICARE AND MEDICAID SERVICES

Clinical Laboratory Improvement Amendments
7500 Security Boulevard
Baltimore MD 21244-1850
877-267-2323
http://cms.hhs.gov/clia/

DOCUMENTATION SYSTEMS

CarePoint, Inc.
215 East Bay Street
Suite 304
Charleston, SC 29401
843-853-6999
www.carepoint.com/cpsite/

Diatrends
Overlook Software, Inc.
1002 N. Church Street, Suite 400
Greensboro, NC 27401-1440
336-274-0066
www.overlooksoftware.com

CMS
The Clinical Management System
Pfizer Health Solutions, Inc.
2400 Broadway, Suite 500
Santa Monica, CA 90404-3030
866-PHS-2002 or 866-747-2002
www.pfizerhealthsolutions.com

Internet Resources for Diabetes

GENERAL

American Diabetes Association
www.diabetes.org

Juvenile Diabetes Research Foundation
www.jdrf.org

International Diabetes Institute
www.diabetes.com.au

Joslin Center
www.joslin.harvard.edu

Diabetes 123
www.diabetes123.com

Children with Diabetes Foundation
www.cwdfoundation.org

HEALTH PROFESSIONALS

American Diabetes Association
www.diabetes.org

Diabetes Care – ADA journal
http://care.diabetesjournals.org

American Association of Clinical Endocrinologists
www.aace.com

American Association of Diabetes Educators
www.aadenet.org

National Institute of Diabetes & Digestive & Kidney Diseases
www.niddk.nih.gov

National Diabetes Education Program
http://ndep.nih.gov

CDC Diabetes Public Health Resource
www.cdc.gov/diabetes

Michigan Diabetes Research and Training Center
www.med.umich.edu/mdrtc/

COMPLICATIONS

FOOT CARE
American Podiatric Medical Association
www.apma.org

EYE HEALTH
National Eye Institute
www.nei.nih.gov

VASCULAR COMPLICATIONS
American Heart Association
www.americanheart.org

National Cholesterol Education Program
www.nhlbi.nih.gov/about/ncep/index.htm

DIET AND EXERCISE

American Heart Association – *diet information*
www.deliciousdecisions.org

Diabetes Exercise and Sports Association
www.diabetes-exercise.org

References

1. Mokdad AH, Bowman BA, Ford ES, et al. The continuing epidemics of obesity and diabetes in the United States. *JAMA.* 2001;286:1195-200.

2. Mokdad AH, Ford ES, Bowman BA, et al. Diabetes trends in the U.S.: 1990-1998. *Diabetes Care.* 2000;23:1278-83.

3. American Diabetes Association. Economic consequences of diabetes mellitus in the U.S. in 1997. *Diabetes Care.* 1998;21:296-309.

4. American Diabetes Association. Position Statement: Diabetic Nephropathy. *Diabetes Care.* 1997;20:S24-7.

5. O'Brien JA, Shomphe LA, Kavanagh PL, et al. Direct medical costs of complications resulting from Type 2 Diabetes in the U.S. *Diabetes Care.* 1998;21:1122-8.

6. The Diabetes Control and Complications Trial Research Group. The effect of intensive treatment of diabetes on the development and progression of long-term complications in insulin-dependent diabetes mellitus. *N Engl J Med.* 1993;329:977-86.

7. UK Prospective Diabetes Study Group. Intensive blood-glucose control with sulphonylureas or insulin compared with conventional treatment and risk of complications in patients with Type 2 diabetes (UKPDS 33). *Lancet.* 1998;352:837-53.

8. Gilmer TP, Manning WG, O'Connor PJ, et al. The cost to health plans of poor glycemic control. *Diabetes Care.* 1997;20:1847-53.

9. Menzin J, Langley-Hawthorne C, Friedman M, et al. Potential short-term economic benefits of improved glycemic control. *Diabetes Care.* 2001;24:51-5.

10. Wagner EH, Sandhu N, Newton KM, et al. Effect of improved glycemic control on health care costs and utilization. *JAMA.* 2001;285:182-9.

11. Rubin RJ, Dietrich KA, Hawk AD. Clinical and economic impact of implementing a comprehensive diabetes management program in managed care. *J Clin Endocrinol Metab.* 1998;83:2635-42.

12. Sikka R, Sutton DR, Waters J, et al. Renal assessment practices and the effect of nurse case management of health maintenance organization patients with diabetes. *Diabetes Care.* 1999;22:1-6.

13. Piette JD, Mah CA, McPhee SJ, et al. Use of automated telephone disease management calls in an ethnically diverse sample of low-income patients with diabetes. *Diabetes Care.* 1999;22:1302-9.

14. Van Veldhuizen-Scott MK, Widmer LB, Stacey SA, et al. Developing and implementing a pharmaceutical care model in an ambulatory care setting for patients with diabetes. *Diabetes Educ.* 1995;21:117-23.

15. Fincham JE, Lofholm PW. Saving money and saving lives: pharmacist care for diabetes patients. *Am Pharm.* March 1998:49-52.

16. Coast-Senior EA, Droner BA, Kelley CL, et al. Management of patients with Type 2 Diabetes by pharmacists in primary care clinics. *Ann Pharmacother.* 1998;32:636-41.

17. Gong C, Hasson NK, Lum BL. Impact of a diabetes disease management clinic on the total glycosolated hemoglobin of patients with Type 2 Diabetes Mellitus. *J Manag Care Pharm.* 1999;5:511-5.

18. Cranor CW, Christensen DB. The Asheville Project: Short-term outcomes of a community pharmacy diabetes care program. *J Am Pharm Assoc.* 2003;43:149-59.

19. Cranor CW, Butning BA, Christensen DB. The Asheville Project: Long-term clinical and economic outcomes of a community pharmacy diabetes care program. *J Am Pharm Assoc.* 2003;43:173-84.

20. Berringer R, Shibley MCH, Cary CC, et al. Outcomes of a community pharmacy-based diabetes monitoring program. *J Am Pharm Assoc.* 1999;39:791-7.

21. Baran RW, Crumlish K, Patterson H, et al. Improving outcomes of community-dwelling older patients with diabetes through patient counseling. *Am J Health Syst Pharm.* 1999;56:1535-9.

22. Irons BK, Lenz RJ, Anderson SL, et al. A retrospective cohort analysis of the clinical effectiveness of a physician-pharmacist collaborative drug therapy management diabetes clinic. *Pharmacotherapy* 2002;22:1294-300.

23. Davidson MB, Karlan VJ, Hair TL. Effect of a pharmacist-managed diabetes care program in a free medical clinic. *Am J Med Qual.* 2000;15:137-42.

24. Jaber LA, Halapy H, Fernet M, et al. Evaluation of a pharmaceutical care model on diabetes management. *Ann Pharmacother.* 1996;30:238-43.

25. Gerber RA, Liu G, McCombs JS. Impact of pharmacist consultations provided to patients with diabetes on healthcare costs in a health maintenance organization. *Am J Manag Care.* 1998;4:991-1000.

26. Kelly C, Rodgers PT. Implementation and evaluation of a pharmacist-managed diabetes service. *J Manag Care Pharm.* 2000;6:488-93.

27. Nau DP, Blevins JD, Neal SE. Collaborating with community pharmacists to improve the quality of diabetes care in an IPA-model HMO. *J Manag Care Pharm.* 2001;7:292-6.

28. Nau DP, Ponte CD. The impact of a community pharmacist-based diabetes patient-management program for managed care enrollees. *J Manag Care Pharm.* 2002;8:48-53.

29. American Diabetes Association. Screening for Diabetes (position statement). *Diabetes Care.* 2002;25:21-4.

30. American Diabetes Association. Standards of Medical Care for Patients with Diabetes Mellitus. *Diabetes Care.* 2002;25:33-49.

31. American Diabetes Association. National Standards for Diabetes Self-Management Education. *Diabetes Care.* 2002;25:140-7.

32. American Association of Diabetes Educators. The Scope of Practice for Diabetes Educators and the Standards of Practice for Diabetes Educators. *Diabetes Educ* 2000;26:25-31.

33. National Institute for Standards in Pharmacist Credentialing. DSM Examinations: Standards/Objectives. Available at: http://www.nispcnet.org. Accessed October 20, 2003.

34. McDonough RP, Doucette WR. Developing collaborative working relationships between pharmacists and physicians. *J Am Pharm Assoc.* 2001;41(5):682-92.

35. McDonough RP, Rovers JP, Currie JD, et al. Obstacles to the implementation of pharmaceutical care in the community setting. *J Am Pharm Assoc.* 1998;38(1):87-95.

36. American Pharmaceutical Association. Principles of Practice for Pharmaceutical Care. Washington, D.C.: APhA; 1995. Available at www.aphanet.org. Accessed October 20, 2003.

37. Rosenthal WM. Establishing a pharmacy based laboratory service. *J Am Pharm Assoc.* 2000;40:146-56.

38. Fitzgerald WL. HIPAA Compliance Handbook for Community Pharmacy. Alexandria, VA: National Community Pharmacists Association; 2003.

39. Schwed D, Miall J, Harteker LR. Pharmacy risk-sharing contracts: do's and don'ts. *J Am Pharm Assoc.* 1999;39:775-84.

40. Farris KB, Kumbera P, Halterman T, et al. Outcomes-based pharmacist reimbursement: reimbursing pharmacists for cognitive services. *J Manag Care Pharm.* 2002;5:383-93.

41. Holdford DA. *Marketing for Pharmacists.* Washington, DC: American Pharmaceutical Association; 2003.

42. Basa RP, McLeod B. Evaluation of a diabetes specialty center: structure, process, and outcome. *Patient Educ Couns.* 1995;25:23-9.

43. Petitti DB, Contreras R, Ziel FH, et al. Evaluation of the effect of performance monitoring and feedback on care process, utilization and outcome. *Diabetes Care.* 2000;23:192-6.

Chapter 2

BUSINESS PLANNING TEMPLATE FOR A DIABETES CARE PRACTICE

David Medvedeff

IN THIS CHAPTER:

- What to Include in the Executive Summary
- Needs Assessment
- Expected Outcomes Section
- Marketing and Action Plan Section
- Effective Use of the Business Plan

A Familiar Format

This chapter consists primarily of a business planning template. The template is modeled according to a clinical paper format so that the process is familiar to you. It guides you through a business planning process in which you think through necessary details and follow practical steps while minimizing the time it takes to assemble a meaningful plan. Having a well developed business plan may be essential to:

1. Obtain internal support or approval of your program.
2. Secure external funding for your program.
3. Keep you on track through the implementation process.

1. EXECUTIVE SUMMARY (ABSTRACT)

The Executive Summary, the first section of the business plan, is similar to the "abstract" in a clinical paper. It should be concise, well-written, and insightful so it catches the reader's interest. The Executive Summary should clarify the following:

- The plan's overall vision
- The need for the service
- Benefits to the stakeholders
- Major steps you will take to implement the service
- Your competitive advantage for offering the service

Include a cover sheet that gives your project title, contact information, address, phone number, and e-mail address. See Figure 2-1 for an example of a cover sheet format.

Figure 2-1.
Sample Cover Sheet for a Business Plan

Business Plan:
Diabetes Management Services
at Medvedeff Pharmacy

Contact Information:
David Medvedeff, Pharm.D., MBA
Medvedeff Clinical Services
1234 Florida Highway
Sunny, FL 12345

Telephone: (777) 555-0001
Fax: (777) 555-0101
Email: dm@internet.com

2. LOCAL NEEDS ASSESSMENT (BACKGROUND)

One of the most critical elements of a successful business is to provide a service or product that directly addresses consumers' needs—especially their "unarticulated" needs.

Meeting unarticulated needs of the consumer typically results in overwhelming success. This same principle applies to health care. If you provide innovative services to meet needs the patient is not fully aware of, you are likely to be successful.

One could argue that in today's health care delivery system, an articulated need of the patient would be spending adequate time with a health care professional. Patients often talk about their frustration regarding the little time they actually get to spend with their physician. Because patients do not understand the full capabilities of pharmacists, they are unlikely to articulate the need to schedule appointments with pharmacists. However, consumer surveys indicate that many people want more information about their health and medications. If you recognize this as an opportunity to capitalize on pharmacists' ability to provide health information, you enhance your probability of providing a successful service.

If you think of your business plan as a clinical paper, the Local Needs Assessment corresponds to the "background" section. Typically, this section of a study discusses why the study is being conducted and what literature is available to support treatment options. The Local Needs Assessment should be applied in much the same way. You should address the following:

- What diabetes services are currently being offered in your community?
- Who is offering these services? What are the specific entities and organizations?
- Who will benefit from your new services?

See Form 8 in the Appendix for a checklist to help you conduct a succinct needs assessment for diabetes care services. Additional information on conducting a needs assessment is provided in Chapter 1, page 11.

3. EXPECTED OUTCOMES OF THE DIABETES PATIENT CARE SERVICE (HYPOTHESES)

Just as you have "hypotheses" in a clinical study, you should have Expected Outcomes from your practice. In other words, you need to know your goals.

Based on your needs assessment information in Form 8, the next step is to identify goals that are important to each stakeholder in the diabetes care service. Some potential stakeholders include the following:

- Patients
- Pharmacists in your practice site
- Diabetes Education Centers in your community
- Physicians
- Employers
- Third-party payers

You must identify goals from the perspective of each stakeholder group. Each group's goals will be different. "ECHO" is a good model to follow as you think through these goals. "E" stands for economic outcomes; "C" for clinical outcomes; and "H" for humanistic outcomes. Table 2-1 provides potential goals in each ECHO category for your practice setting and community.

Using the table as a guide, consider the stakeholder needs unique to your practice setting and community. Prepare a bulleted list of goals for your business plan from the perspective of each stakeholder group, which you can place in the Expected Outcomes section.

4. MARKETING AND ACTION PLAN FOR ESTABLISHING DIABETES CARE SERVICES FOR SELF-INSURED EMPLOYERS/PAYERS (METHODS)

This section of the business plan is similar to the "methods" section in a clinical paper. It outlines the steps required to meet the expected outcomes you identified after conducting your needs assessment. You need a plan to market your diabetes care service as well as an action plan for putting the necessary components in place for a sustainable service.

To market your diabetes services you must first define your "product." In other words, what are the components of your diabetes services and how will they be provided? The key components should be based on the opportunities within your community as discovered in your needs assessment. Your business plan should contain a description of the services, written on a level understandable to the readers (remembering that not all readers may be health care professionals).

Once your services have been defined, it is important to determine how payment for

TABLE 2-1. Sample Goals for Various Stakeholders

Stakeholder Group	Economic Goals	Clinical Goals	Humanistic Goals
Patients	Reduced out-of-pocket costs (waived copays, free meters)	Reduced HbA1c levels, improved lipid profiles, reduced weight, reduced foot sores	Better satisfaction with care, enhanced quality of life
Pharmacists	Payment for diabetes care services	Increased patient medication and blood glucose monitoring adherence	Improved job satisfaction
Diabetes Education Center	Payment for diabetes education programs	Improved nutrition, exercise, and stress management	Enhanced follow-up for patient education
Physicians	Increased preventive care for diabetes; decreased urgent care visits	Patients following individualized care plans; better glycemic control	Continuity of care for people with diabetes
Employers	Reduced total health care costs for employees with diabetes	Improved HEDIS* scores; reduced long-term complications	Reduced sick days for people with diabetes; increased satisfaction with health benefits
Third-Party Payers	Decreased hospital visits leading to lower total costs	Data on HbA1c levels, and improved HEDIS* scores	Improved health plan satisfaction for people with diabetes

*The Health Plan Employer Data and Information Set (HEDIS) is a set of standardized measures for health care purchasers and consumers that is used to assess performance of managed care organizations. More information about the HEDIS measures is available from the National Committee for Quality Assurance (NCQA) at www.ncqa.org.

the services will be obtained. The strategy that has proven most successful for obtaining payment for pharmacist diabetes care services is based on the Asheville Project.[1] Within the Asheville Project, self-insured employers teamed with community pharmacists to improve diabetes self-management skills for their employees. The pharmacists were paid to provide diabetes education and care management to employees of the City of Asheville and of a large health care system. They helped diabetes patients achieve better health while lowering the total costs of care for the employers. The CD-ROM that accompanies this book includes a Power Point presentation about the Asheville Project and its results, which you can use to help sell your program to employers and payers in your community. It's an effective example of the difference that pharmacists' efforts can make in patient outcomes.

Make a list of local business owners and human resource benefit managers whom you can contact when you are ready to implement your service. When approaching larger employers, it may be more effective to present your concept in collaboration with other pharmacists in your community who are also interested in providing this service. Employers are generally interested in having a network of providers so their employees have a choice of locations at which to receive services.

The list below provides the action steps generally necessary to implement a program similar to the Asheville Project in your community. Form 9 in Appendix A, "Action Planning Timeline and Responsibilities Chart," also includes these steps and provides space for you to identify the person responsible for each step, as well as the target dates for completion.

- Establish a network of diabetes care pharmacists who have the necessary skills, consultation areas, and commitment to provide the services.
- Adopt care processes and outcome monitoring measures that are standardized across all network pharmacies.
- Develop collaborative relationships with physicians and gain support for your services.
- Promote diabetes care services to local self-insured providers and obtain commitment for payment.
- Develop a payment schedule and processes to receive payment for services.
- Work with the employer(s) to establish processes for enrolling employees and tracking economic outcomes.

Work on each of the above steps simultaneously. Some components may already be in place, thus allowing you to focus on tasks that are not yet finished. Completing Form 9 will generate a timeline and a plan for putting in place each component of your diabetes patient care service.

Use the accounting spreadsheets on the CD-ROM (and reproduced as Forms 10-12 in Appendix A at the end of this book) to determine the costs of operating the diabetes service and the revenue required to achieve economic success.

5. EVALUATING POTENTIAL SUCCESS OF THE BUSINESS PLAN (FINDINGS, LIMITATIONS, AND CONCLUSIONS)

The final step in completing your business plan is to take a critical look at where you expect to succeed and where you find shortcomings, as in the final section of a clinical paper, which addresses "findings, limitations, and conclusions." A good way to identify potential areas of success and improvement is to analyze your strengths, weaknesses, opportunities, and threats, commonly known as a "SWOT Analysis." Based on the results of this structured analysis you can develop strategies for taking advantage of your strengths and opportunities and overcoming your weaknesses and threats.

A good starting point for the SWOT analysis is to review the previous sections of the business plan. Look over each section and categorize the major items in your plan into one of the four quadrants on the chart (see Chapter 1, page 11). Strengths and weaknesses are items that are under direct control within your practice site; opportunities and threats are outside forces that you have limited ability to influence.

The challenge now is to develop strategies to take advantage of your strengths and opportunities and action steps for overcoming your weaknesses and threats. Because you can't focus on everything, identify three strategies for emphasizing your program's strengths and three action steps to overcome the most significant barriers. Get input from your staff to develop this list. Post it where everyone can see it to maintain their focus on these items.

6. APPENDIX

Your appendix can include additional attachments to the business plan. For example:

- **Organizational structure of the service.** Who's in charge and what other roles are involved?
- **Key people.** Résumés and background information for each person involved, including their training and additional certification in the area of diabetes.

Effective Use of the Business Plan

The business plan should strike a balance between detail and succinctness. It needs to convey important information to the reader without providing so much detail that the main points are lost. However, there should be enough information in the plan (e.g., assumptions underlying your projected revenue) for the reader to make an informed decision regarding your plan.

It may be useful to have one or two other people read your plan to be sure it is clear and effective before you submit it for approval. If you are seeking external funds for a new business venture, you may also want to consult with a local office of the U.S. Small Business Administration (www.sba.gov), which can provide feedback on your business plan.

A well-thought-out plan is the key to success for your new services. The planning process will help you identify the opportunities and threats to your new services, and your written plan will help to keep you on track through the implementation and evaluation of your new services. The plan should also be updated as new opportunities arise or as your experience with the service leads you to program improvements.

References

1. Garrett DG, Martin LA. The Asheville Project: Participants' perceptions of factors contributing to the success of a patient self-management diabetes program. *J Am Pharm Assoc.* 2003;43:185-90.

Chapter 3

BUILDING A QUALITY IMPROVEMENT PROGRAM FOR PHARMACY-BASED DIABETES SERVICES

David Nau and Virginia Scott

IN THIS CHAPTER:
- Basics of Quality Improvement
- Evaluating Quality of Care
- Performance Indicators
- Organizing the QI Team
- Causes of Process Variation
- Sustaining the QI Program

The Basics of Quality Improvement

Quality is important in pharmacy service. Most pharmacists care about their patients and seek to provide safe, useful services. The American Pharmaceutical Association Code of Ethics for pharmacists addresses the pharmacist's obligation to the well-being of the patient and community, and the *National Association of Boards of Pharmacy Model State Pharmacy Act and Model Rules* notes the pharmacist's responsibility for the safety of pharmaceutical services.[1,2]

Though they accept this responsibility, few community pharmacists use systematic methods to evaluate and improve the quality of their services. Like many health care providers, we pharmacists often rely on our own intuition or informal feedback from patients to evaluate the quality of our care. Unfortunately, our perceptions of how well we perform don't always match our patients' impressions or actual performance data.[3,4] Integrating the philosophies and process of quality improvement (QI) into the practice of pharmacy may be the key to optimizing the quality of care we provide.

In recent years, the quality of care provided by health care professionals has come under increased scrutiny. In 1999, the Institute of Medicine report on medical errors heightened the public's awareness of quality-related problems in hospitals.[5] This report caused many hospitals to more seriously address the way in which the philosophy of quality improvement had been integrated into their daily operations. Other organizations such as the Joint Commission for the Accreditation of Healthcare Organizations (JCAHO), the National Committee for Quality Assurance (NCQA), the Foundation for Accountability (FACCT), the Automotive Industry Action Group (AIAG), Public Citizen, and the Leapfrog Group have all pushed for greater attention to health care quality in recent years. Several states have also implemented requirements for pharmacies to have quality assurance and/or quality improvement processes.[6]

When implementing specialized patient care programs such as diabetes patient management services, quality of care is especially important. Quality improvement processes for diabetes care have been shown to enhance care in ambulatory settings.[7-9] The American Diabetes Association National Standards for Diabetes Self-Management Education (DSME) recognizes the importance of quality improvement through Standard 10: "The DSME entity will utilize a continuous quality improvement process to evaluate the effectiveness of the education experience provided, and determine opportunities for improvement."[10] Therefore, any DSME program that seeks ADA recognition will need a quality improvement process.

WHAT IS QUALITY IMPROVEMENT?

Practitioners are sometimes confused when faced with the myriad of quality-related acronyms being used today, such as CQI, QI, QA, TQM, SPC, and PDCA. Things become even murkier when you add the many different quality-related philosophies—kaizen, zero-defects, quality circles, organizational learning, process re-engineering—and the distinctions between quality improvement, quality assurance, and quality control are sometimes blurry, as well.

Confusion may arise from the differing terminology and philosophies of quality gurus such as W. Edwards Deming, Walter Shewhart, Philip Crosby, Joseph Juran, and Armand Feigenbaum, and from the evolution of quality-related terminology in health care systems driven by JCAHO, NCQA and others.

Quality improvement can generally be characterized by certain attributes, which are listed in the box on page 32. The quality improvement process is typically implemented via the PDCA (Shewhart) Cycle (see Figure 3-1), also called the Deming Cycle (although

Figure 3-1.
The Shewhart or Deming Cycle for Quality Improvement

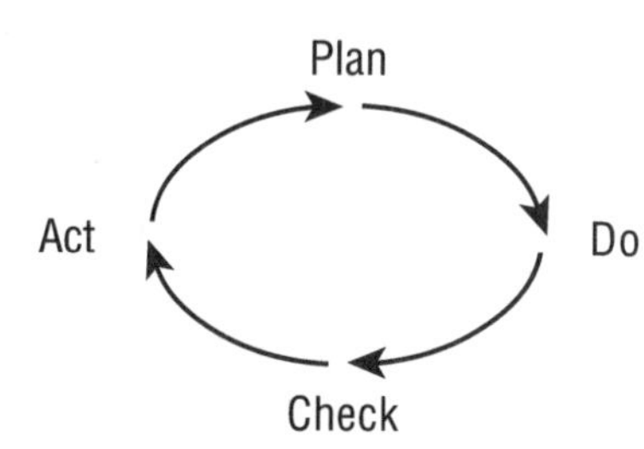

Deming referred to it as the Shewhart Cycle).[11,12] This cyclical process involves four key elements: Plan, Do, Check, Act.

In a diabetes patient-management service (DPMS), *Plan* would entail designing a new approach for providing the DPMS that leads to an improvement in quality. This approach would include guidelines or procedures for how care will be provided, and also plans for how the care process will be evaluated. The *Do* step in the cycle concerns the implementation of the new plan, while *Check* refers to an objective evaluation of the plan. Once we have checked the performance of our new plan, we can *Act* upon the performance data to standardize the new plan (assuming that it led to significant improvement) or we can further revise the existing plan and repeat the PDCA cycle.

An extension of the Shewhart cycle is called FOCUS-PDCA.[13] This approach was developed by the Hospital Corporation of America to facilitate quality improvement efforts in their hospitals. The first step of FOCUS-PDCA is to *Find* the process that will be targeted for improvement (e.g., the DPMS enrollment process). The second step is to *Organize* a team to study the problem (e.g., pharmacists, technicians, patients, and other providers). Next, we *Clarify* the team's understanding of the process (i.e., ensure that everyone has a common understanding of how the care process is actually being carried out, perhaps through the use of a flow diagram). Then, we seek to *Understand* the root causes of variation in performance (i.e., identify problems—such as a poorly designed workflow, inadequate training, or unclear roles—and determine why they occur). Finally, we *Select* the parts of the structure or process to change. Once we have selected the target for change, we can formulate a new *Plan* for how the process will change and then continue the PDCA cycle through the *Do, Check,* and *Act* steps.

Quality Improvement Is:

- **Prospective**—forward-thinking; always looking for better ways to provide care.
- **Continuous**—a standard element of practice rather than a one-time effort.
- **Team-oriented**—a collaborative effort of all employees and management; recognizes the unique and valuable knowledge of each team member.
- **Nonpunitive**—employees should be rewarded for identifying problems/mistakes and not be fearful of discussing operational problems.
- **Systems-oriented**—focus of improvement efforts is on the process or system of care rather than the elimination of "bad" employees.
- **Customer-focused**—all team members are focused on fulfilling the needs of the customer (e.g., patient, physician, other team members).
- **Data-driven**—evaluates performance based on objective data.

EVALUATING THE QUALITY OF CARE

One of the most challenging elements of quality improvement is measuring the quality of care. Health care quality has frequently been evaluated using the framework established by Avedis Donabedian, which subdivides medical care quality into three parts: Structure, Process, and Outcome.[14]

The Donabedian framework can also be used to evaluate the quality of pharmaceutical care.[15] In pharmaceutical terms *Structure* refers to the characteristics of providers, the tools and resources at their disposal, and the physical or organizational settings in which they work. Examples include professional licensure or certification, computer systems for tracking patient information, patient counseling areas, and human resource policies. The elements of structure create the environment for care. These structural elements may be necessary to provide optimal care, but their presence does not ensure optimal care.

Process refers to the set of activities that occur between patient and provider, encompassing the services and products that we provide to patients as well as the manner in which the services are provided. Experts often group the specific elements of care processes within two domains: technical or interpersonal.[15] The technical domain of pharmaceutical care may include gathering patient information, entering prescription information into computers, reviewing patient profiles, checking prescription labels, evaluating a patient's laboratory results, identifying and resolving potential drug-related problems, and answering patient questions. The interpersonal domain of pharmaceutical care includes the ability of the pharmacist to express empathy, listen attentively, and develop a caring relationship with the patient.

Process of care is often the primary focus of our quality improvement efforts as we strive to *Do* what is best for our patients. Care processes can be directly evaluated by using the norms or standards that exist across the health care system (e.g., what is commonly accepted as good care), or indirectly by determining their impact on outcomes.[14,15,16]

The term *outcomes* was originally defined by Donabedian as "a change in a patient's current and future health status that can be attributed to antecedent health care."[14] Lohr also characterized outcomes in terms of the consequences of medical care for patients (death, disability, disease, discomfort, and dissatisfaction).[17] In later years, the use of this term has broadened to encompass the economic, clinical, and humanistic consequences of health care processes (ECHO Model).[18] Within the ECHO model, outcomes may include economic consequences (e.g., costs of care), clinical measures or endpoints (e.g., blood pressure, HbA1c, pain, mortality), and humanistic issues (patient satisfaction or health-related quality of life).

Outcomes are sometimes classified as *intermediate* or *long-term.* This terminology results from seeing the link between process and numerous outcomes as a causal chain of events.[14,16] Intermediate outcomes may occur between the health care process and long-term, or ultimate outcomes. For example, providing pharmacist counseling services regarding the appropriate use of blood glucose meters (the process) will lead to better adherence with the meter (an intermediate outcome) which leads to more appropriate adjustments of medications (another intermediate outcome) that leads to better glycemic control (another intermediate outcome) that will in turn lead to better health-related quality of life (the long-term outcome). Thus, when evaluating the linkage of the pharmaceutical care *process* with long-term pharmaceutical care *outcomes*, it may be useful to identify potential intermediate outcomes along the causal path between the process and long-term outcomes.[16]

PERFORMANCE INDICATORS

Within the Shewhart cycle for continuous quality improvement (Plan-Do-Check-Act), quality is often *checked* through the use of performance indicators.[19] These indicators are measures or screens for quality, and can focus on either structure, process, or outcomes. Typically, they measure specific functions within a process or outcomes known to be associated with the process. Although one might think that outcomes are the ideal indicator of health care performance, they are often more difficult to measure than specific health care functions and may not always be directly, or independently, caused by the process of interest. Process indicators are useful for quality improvement in the circumstances outlined in the box below.

Process Indicators Are Useful When:

- Outcome is difficult to measure.
- Outcome is far removed in time from the process.
- Outcome is influenced by many factors other than the process.
- Outcome is not responsive to change in the process.

Therefore, if one wanted to improve the quality of pharmaceutical care for persons with diabetes, it may be more useful to assess the appropriateness of adjustments in insulin doses than to measure the rate of hospitalizations over a 5-year period for patients in the pharmaceutical care program. This is not to suggest that evaluating outcomes is unwise. If outcomes can be directly linked to the process and also can be evaluated in a timely, efficient, and reliable manner, they become powerful tools for quality improvement.

Indicators should be selected on the basis of their usefulness to your quality improvement efforts. The indicator should help determine where potential problems are occurring within the process that you control. For example, it may be useful to know that only 30% of your patients reported that they were provided with adequate answers to their questions about medications. You can change the way you provide drug-related information to your patients. However, it would not be as helpful to know that only 30% of your patients with diabetes had received a microalbumin test if you do not control when that test is ordered.

Indicators for ongoing performance assessment are best constructed as a proportion, percentage, or ratio, rather than as raw counts. The denominator within the ratio should be the total number of persons within the target population, while the numerator should be the number of persons who received (or failed to receive) the desired test, or who achieved a specified goal. For example, if we wanted to construct an indicator for medication errors, the numerator would be the number of medication errors within a defined time period and the denominator would be the total number of error opportunities (e.g., number of prescriptions filled) during the same time period. This facilitates the comparison of error rates over time, even as prescription volume fluctuates.

It will also be necessary to provide definitions for any variables that are not intuitive. *Medication error* means different things to different people, so if one wanted to construct an indicator for medication errors, it would be necessary to inform your staff what constitutes an error. You should also identify inclusion or exclusion criteria.

For diabetes-related indicators, we need to decide whether to combine data for all patients with diabetes mellitus, or to subdivide the analyses for Type 1 and Type 2 diabetes. Other questions include: What about gestational diabetes? Do we include people of all ages? Do we include only those who attended all diabetes education sessions, or anyone who completed even a portion of the program? The answers to these questions may depend upon the particular indicator. The key is to compare "apples to apples." If, for example, the standard for HbA1c testing is different for persons with gestational diabetes as compared to Type 1 or Type 2 diabetes mellitus, then you would not want to combine HbA1c data from all these patients into a single indicator.

In order to judge the quality of performance from the indicator data, it will be necessary to have a frame of reference. Thus, your current performance data can be compared to your previous performance (i.e., did we improve over time) or can be compared to an external criterion or standard (i.e., did we exceed the minimal standards).[3,13] Both comparisons can be useful.

For example, you could track the proportion of your patients who reached the target HbA1c over the past 2 years (e.g., 45% of patients last year versus 62% of patients this year). However, it is less clear whether 62% of patients reaching the target is considered good, fair, or poor performance. To determine this, we could compare our "success" rate to that of other programs. If the latest data from surrounding health plans indicates that 60% of their enrollees with diabetes have achieved the same target for HbA1c, then we could assert that our performance is at least as good as the standard. Ideally, your goal will be to continually improve your success rate, regardless of the minimal standard.

Implementing a Quality Improvement Program for Pharmacy-Based Care

IDENTIFY THE PROCESS TO IMPROVE

The first step in the FOCUS-PDCA cycle is to identify the process to improve. Although we may not think of our clinical practice as a "process," we often follow a logical sequence of steps in providing patient education and monitoring services. Diabetes care could involve numerous processes that include patient enrollment, scheduling, physical assessment, patient education (with subprocesses on glucose meter instruction, insulin injection training, etc), or drug-therapy modification.

Selecting the process for improvement may result from identifying problems (or potential problems) in your practice, or simply because the process is very important to the success of your program. Key factors in the selection are that the process must be observable, measurable, and have clearly defined boundaries. When choosing a process to improve, it may be helpful to ask yourself the questions in the box above right.[20] If this is your first foray into quality improvement, it may be best to select a process that is simple, small, and totally controlled by your pharmacy before attempting to improve more complex processes involving other health care providers.

Process Improvement Selection

When selecting a process for improvement, ask the following questions:

- Can the process be defined?
- Does the problem occur frequently?
- Is the problem well-known to all who work within the process?
- Will people appreciate it if the process is improved?
- Is there a good chance of success in improving the process?
- Will little or no outside help be needed to implement the changes?
- Is this really a process improvement effort or an attempt to impose a predetermined solution to a problem?

ORGANIZE THE QI TEAM

After the process is selected, the QI team should be organized. When selecting your team, you must determine the size, identify the members and team leader, write the objective for process improvement and team statement, and develop the team's ground rules and effectiveness guidelines.

Team Size and Structure

Team size should range from three to seven members. Teams larger than seven (especially those of 10 or more) tend to be inefficient. Team members should be selected from the individuals working in the diabetes patient management service. Individuals who may be included are the pharmacy manager or owner, staff pharmacists, certified diabetes educators, pharmacy technicians, dietitians, physicians, or other individuals involved in the service.

Individuals may volunteer to serve on the team or be selected by management. Ideally, you should choose individuals who have good interpersonal communication skills, problem-solving and decision-making skills, knowledge of the process, a willingness to accept the concepts of QI, and the ability to accept the responsibility of team membership.

Within an organization, there may be several QI teams depending on the process or processes selected for improvement. For example, the team examining the process for dispensing medications to patients with diabetes may be different from the team addressing the process of patient monitoring for clinical parameters such as glucose levels, blood pressure, and other values or tests.

A team leader is selected from the team members by management or elected by the other members. Before accepting the team leader role, the individual selected should understand her responsibilities. Her tasks will include scheduling and running the meetings and interacting with management. The leader will work with management to determine how the team's time will be used, the timeline for completing the improvement process, the procedure for communicating the teams' recommendations, the team's authority for decision-making, and also to secure resources needed by the team.

Process Improvement Objective

At the first meeting of the team, a process improvement objective should be developed for the purpose of keeping the team focused. The objective states what needs to be improved in the process or the expected results from changes in the process. An example of a process improvement objective for the selected process of monitoring patients with diabetes is "To improve the successful outcomes of patients with diabetes, adherence to follow-up visits should be greater than 90%."

Team Statement

The team should develop a written team statement. This information may be in a narrative format or in a form such as the "Quality Improvement Team Statement"[20] that appears as Form 13 in Appendix A.

The team statement should consist of three sections: process definition, team leadership, and team definition. The process definition section should identify the process being examined, describe the team's boundaries, and state the process improvement objective. Names of all team members and the leader should be noted under team leadership. The last section, team definition, focuses on the procedures identified for conducting team meetings, such as the frequency of meetings, start/stop times, decision-making authority, reporting requirements, or other issues.

Ground Rules

Ground rules should be established for the team meetings and team members. The team meeting ground rules are defined by the team members. These should include the tracking of assignments, selection of a recorder for team meetings, method for making decisions such as majority or consensus, and a method for keeping members focused on the future process rather than "how things were done" in the past.

The team leader should establish ground rules for the team members. These may include an attendance policy, standard for promptness to meetings, and time line for completion of assignments. The leader also encourages active listening, free communication, and courtesy to other members (such as one person speaking at a time and no side conversations).

Effective Team Meetings

Effective meetings are important for the team's success. In addition to following the meeting ground rules suggested above, several other strategies enhance the effectiveness and efficiency of meetings. These strategies include using an agenda, publishing the agenda prior to the meeting, recording minutes of team meetings, and distributing information to team members prior to the meeting.

CLARIFICATION OF THE PROCESS

Team members must clarify the current process before identifying methods to improve that process. To identify the steps within a given process, it may be helpful to use a "Work Process Flow Chart" as shown in Figure 3-2. The flow chart should be created with the input of all team members to ensure that everyone has a common understanding of the process. Sometimes, the construction of the flow chart uncovers inconsistencies or uncertainties in how the process is carried out. Prior to recording the agreed-upon workflow, it may be best to write each step of the process on a Post-It note. These notes attach easily to a board or wall and can be moved to create your final work process.

Here's an example to help you understand this step in the FOCUS-PDCA Cycle. The process being examined is "enrollment of patients in the diabetes care program." The QI team consists of a pharmacist, pharmacy technician, physician, and nurse. The team begins by identifying all the possible entry points for patients into the system. Most likely, they will come up with two means of identifying newly diagnosed patients for enrollment; for example, when the patient presents a prescription at the pharmacy, or when the physician makes the diagnosis. For the sake of efficiency, they may choose to focus on the process of enrollment based on the presentation of a new diabetes prescription at the pharmacy.

Figure 3-2.
Example of Flow Chart for Obtaining Statement of Medical Necessity (SMN)

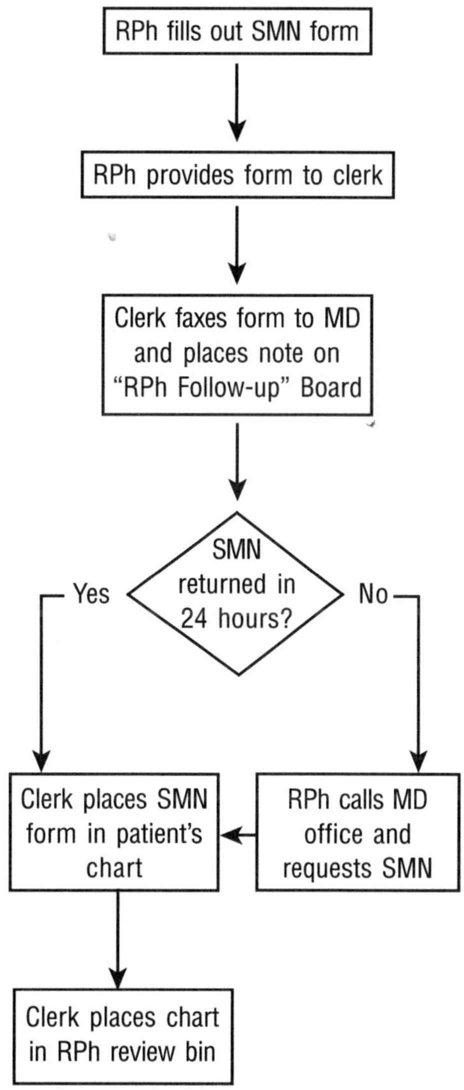

The team would then identify all of the steps in the process for enrollment of this patient. These may include:

1. The technician alerts the pharmacist that a new diabetes prescription was received.
2. The pharmacist determines if the patient is eligible for participation.
3. The pharmacist informs the patient of the availability of the diabetes care program.
4. The pharmacist obtains agreement from the patient to participate.
5. The pharmacist sends a fax to the physician's office to obtain a referral and to determine the manner in which the physician wishes to exchange information regarding the patient.
6. The receptionist at the physician's office places the referral form in the "urgent message" box at the physician's office.
7. The physician reviews and signs the referral request.
8. The receptionist faxes the completed referral form to the pharmacy.
9. The pharmacist contacts the patient to schedule an appointment. Additional detail can be added to the process flow sheet once the basic steps are agreed upon.

Clarification of each step within the process is important for the purpose of understanding and defining variations. It may be useful to ask the following questions for each step: Where does it take place? When does it occur? Who is involved? What training, procedures, policies, equipment, and facilities are involved? What performance standards should be used? What tools or information are needed?[20] The team should reach agreement on the answers to these questions so that a common understanding of the workflow is maintained.

UNDERSTAND CAUSES OF PROCESS VARIATION

The fourth step in the FOCUS-PDCA Cycle is to understand the causes of process variation. For each activity in the process, the team performs a root cause analysis. The "root cause" is the source from which the variation originates. Thus, a deviation in the process may result from one or multiple "root causes."

In the previous example, you might have determined that numerous individuals were getting new prescriptions filled for diabetes medications without being informed about the diabetes care program. The team wants to identify all of the possible reasons that the patients are not being informed of the program, and they may use an idea-generating technique like brainstorming to encourage all team members to contribute. When brainstorming, team members come up with ideas in a free flow fashion, and all ideas are acceptable. The ideas may be specific or vague. The goal is to generate as many ideas as possible, and team members are encouraged to build on the ideas of others.

The team might identify many potential causes for the problem. They might include: the technician was not informed that she should be flagging the new diabetes prescriptions; the technician is distracted by many other responsibilities; the technician verbally informed the pharmacist, but the pharmacist forgot to talk with the patient; the patient was not in the store at the time the new prescription was telephoned to the pharmacy; and the pharmacists had changed shifts before the patient arrived.

After the team identifies many possible root causes for the problem, they may begin to rank the problems in order of perceived frequency, or they could collect data to systematically assess this. Once the most common causes of the problem are identified, the PDCA Cycle can be used to improve the system.

THE PDCA CYCLE

Plan and Do

The PDCA cycle is Plan, Do, Check, and Act. The team *plans* changes in the process to correct the variation. For the previous example, the plan might be to attach a preprinted slip of paper to the prescription container that indicates that the patient should be informed of the diabetes care program. Next, employees will implement or *do* the changes as recommended to correct system variations. Prior to implementing the change, it is important to make sure that everyone involved in the dispensing process is informed of the new plan.

Check

In order to determine whether the new process has led to improvements, it would be best to systematically measure or *check* the impact of the improvement (rather than relying only on your "gut" feeling). This is often done through the use of performance indicators. As described previously, indicators are quantitative measures of key elements in your process.

Numerous organizations have developed indicator systems for diabetes care. For example, the National Committee for Quality Assurance (NCQA) has developed a set of indicators for managed care organizations called the HealthPlan Employer Data and Information Set (HEDIS).[21] HEDIS contains "effectiveness-of-care" indicators for numerous disease states including diabetes mellitus. The Comprehensive Diabetes Care indicator set is described in the box below. Although these indicators address the clinical management of diabetes, they do not directly address diabetes self-management education (DSME).

Comprehensive Diabetes Care Indicators

The Diabetes Care Indicators estimate the percentage of health plan members with Type 1 and Type 2 diabetes 18-75 years old who during the measurement year:

- Had a glycosolated hemoglobin (HbA1c) test.
- Had poorly controlled HbA1c (HbA1c > 9.5%).
- Had a cholesterol (LDL) test.
- Had an LDL level less than 130 mg/dL.
- Had a microalbumin test.
- Had a dilated eye exam.

The American Association of Diabetes Educators (AADE) has supported the development of the National Diabetes Education Outcomes System (NDEOS).[22] This system offers a framework for the evaluation of DSME at the patient level as well as the program level. Software programs (D-SMART and D-ET) have also been developed to facilitate the collection and analysis of data within the NDEOS framework. The NDEOS hopes that participating diabetes education programs can add their data to a central database that will allow national evaluations of the impact of diabetes education.

For pharmacy-based diabetes patient management services, there are myriad performance indicators that could be utilized. However, it is important to select indicators that reflect the key components of your diabetes care program. If your program provides only medication-related counseling for patients with diabetes, then it does not make sense to evaluate your program based upon the frequency of HbA1c testing of your patients.

However, multidisciplinary programs will typically have a broad mixture of indicators that reflect the performance of the team rather than any individual practitioner. In the preceding example regarding the enrollment of patients in the diabetes care program, an indicator could be constructed to measure the proportion of eligible patients who were offered the opportunity to enroll.

A list of potential diabetes-related performance indicators is listed in Table 3-1. These are just a few of the indicators that could be constructed regarding the education or clinical management of patients with diabetes. To assess the education process, data on patient knowledge, skills, or behavior are often collected via interviews or questionnaires. Data for the clinical management indicators can be collected through a variety of means, depending on the relationships between the pharmacist, physician, laboratories, and patients.

The availability of patient-level data is inherent to the development of program-level indicators. The program-level indicators are typically constructed through the aggregation of patient-specific data, so if you are not tracking whether an individual patient has received an HbA1c test, you would be unable to determine what proportion of your patient population has received this test. Collecting and organizing data for performance indicators can be facilitated through software programs. A review of software for diabetes clinical management can be found in a recent edition of *Diabetes Educator*.[23]

When selecting indicators for diabetes education, it is usually best to identify those that reflect the key educational goals of the program. Indicators pertaining to the process of diabetes education will often be the most useful for quality improvement because they identify whether key actions have been taken by patients and providers (e.g., whether patients have returned for follow-up visits and whether pharmacists have completed a thorough assessment of drug therapy). Outcomes-oriented indicators may be less useful in identifying "opportunities for improvement" since they are often influenced by factors beyond the control of the pharmacist.

For example, the health-related quality of life for diabetes patients may be influenced by age, comorbid conditions, the level of support provided by family members, the prescribing decisions of physicians, the patient's occupation, and numerous other clinical, social, and financial factors. Thus, it may be difficult to evaluate the quality of the diabetes education program based solely on the scores from a measure of health-related quality of life.

Some quality of life measures may be useful in identifying the concerns of your patients and the types of limitations that they experience. However, the use of quality of life instruments for the purposes of program assessment is much more complex. If a clinician hopes to evaluate the impact of a diabetes education program on the quality of life of his/her patients, then it may be best to work with trained researchers to design an evaluation process that will provide a valid assessment of the impact of the program. Many measures can be found in the Quality

TABLE 3-1. Examples of Performance Indicators for Pharmacy-Based Diabetes Education

Indicator	Definition*	Data Source	Comments
Return Visits	Percentage of patients who return for all scheduled appointments/classes during the first 6 months of program.	Patient records and/or clinic schedules.	Exclude patients who were unable to return due to relocation, illness, hospitalization, or injury.
Diabetes Knowledge	Percentage of patients who achieve a passing score on a test of diabetes knowledge.	Questionnaire	A validated test of diabetes knowledge should be administered after completion of educational program.
Blood Glucose Monitoring (BGM)	Percentage of patients who adhere to agreed-upon schedule for BGM.	Patient records, diaries, survey, strip refills	Patient BGM adherence can be tracked via diaries or with meters that allow data to be downloaded to software.
Medication Use	Percentage of patients who adhere to medication regimen.	Rx refill record, patient diary, survey, or pill counts	Indicator could be calculated separately for patients on insulin versus oral drug therapy.
Patient Satisfaction	Percentage of patients who indicate that they are satisfied with each element of the diabetes care program.	Questionnaire	A multidimensional measure should be used to identify patients' satisfaction with each of the key elements of the diabetes care program.
Complete Data	Percentage of patient charts that have a complete set of documentation for each education and monitoring session.	Patient records	The thoroughness of documentation is essential to tracking patient progress and for evaluating the appropriateness of care.

* Definitions presented in this table are examples. The definition of an indicator should be tailored to the design of the diabetes care program, as should inclusion/exclusion criteria and methods for data collection.

of Life Instruments Database.[24] A review of health-related quality of life measurement in diabetes has been provided by Luscombe.[25]

It may be more useful to measure the patients' satisfaction with the pharmacy-based diabetes care program. The most efficient way to collect data on satisfaction is through the use of a brief questionnaire. Several measures of pharmacy satisfaction have been described in the professional literature.[26] While these measures cover many aspects of pharmacy services, some clinicians may want to choose a simple method of evaluating satisfaction that uses only a few questions. A 10-item measure of patients' opinions regarding pharmacy-based diabetes patient management services has been developed by Shibley and colleagues.[27]

Act

Once the data are collected, the team will evaluate it and *Act* on the results. Data are evaluated by comparing past performance to current performance. If the process has not improved, the team restarts the PDCA Cycle by planning other changes, implementing them, checking for improvements, and acting on the results. If the process has improved, the team should determine a date for reevaluation to ensure that performance does not decline over time.

SUSTAINING THE QI PROGRAM

The QI program is sustained by both the staff and management of the organization. Staff commitment comes from both being involved in the QI process and a willingness to make changes recommended by management. The QI team leader must inform all individuals working within the process of the results from the QI effort and the impact of these improvements on patient care. These results may be communicated verbally or in writing with the use of visual aids such as bar, pie, or trend charts; and also tables containing statistical information such as numbers, ratios, and percentages.

The results of the QI team should also be communicated to management. Ultimately, management is responsible for sustaining the QI process. This responsibility comes through the willingness to try the changes recommended by the QI teams, and to provide resources such as training, new equipment, redesigning the workplace and/or other needs. Management should reward and recognize employees committed to quality rather than using punitive action when a deviation occurs. If management is not committed to this process, quality and efficiency within the organization will decline.

In summary, develop a standardized plan for QI, train everyone on the plan, implement the plan 100% of the time, evaluate performance, analyze the data collected, revise the plan if there is deviation from the process, and reward good performance. Implementing continuous quality improvement in your Diabetes Patient Management Service will result in a more effective and efficient service.

References

1. American Pharmacists Association. Code of Ethics for Pharmacists. Available at: http://www.aphanet.org/pharmcare/ethics.html. Accessed October 16, 2003.
2. National Association of Boards of Pharmacy. Model State Pharmacy Act and Model Rules. Available at: http://www.nabp.net. Accessed October 16, 2003
3. Hepler CD. Regulating for outcomes as a systems response to the problem of drug-related morbidity. *J Am Pharm Assoc.* 2001;41:108-15.
4. Davies AR, Ware JE. Involving consumers in quality of care assessment. *Health Aff.* Spring 1988:33-48.
5. IOM Committee on Quality in Health Care in America. *To Err is Human–Building a Safer Health System.* Washington, DC: National Academy Press; 1999.
6. Ukens C. Regulating for outcomes: Is it in your future? *Drug Topics.* September 18, 2000:75-6.
7. Fox CH, Mahoney MC. Improving diabetes preventive care in a family practice residency program: a case study in continuous quality improvement. *Fam Med.* 1998;30:441-5.
8. O'Connor PJ, Rush WA, Peterson J, et al. Continuous quality improvement can improve glycemic control for HMO patients with diabetes. *Arch Fam Med.* 1996;5:502-6.
9. Petitti DB, Contreras R, Ziel FH, et al. Evaluation of the effect of performance monitoring and feedback on care process, utilization and outcome. *Diabetes Care.* 2000;23:192-6.
10. American Diabetes Association. National Standards for Diabetes Self-Management Education. *Diabetes Care.* 2001; 24:S126-33.
11. Deming WE. *Out of the Crisis.* Cambridge, MA: Massachusetts Institute of Technology, Center for Advanced Engineering Study; 1986.
12. Deming WE. *The New Economics for Industry, Education, Government.* Cambridge, MA: Massachusetts Institute of Technology, Center for Advanced Engineering Study; 1993.
13. McLaughlin CP, Kaluzny AD. *Continuous Quality Improvement in Health Care.* 2nd ed. Gaithersburg, MD: Aspen Publishers Inc; 1999.
14. Donabedian A. Explorations in quality assessment and monitoring. In: *The Definition of Quality and Approaches to Its Assessment.* Ann Arbor, MI: Health Administration Press; 1980:79-128.
15. Farris KB, Kirking DM. Assessing the quality of pharmaceutical care II: application of concepts of quality assessment from medical care. *Ann Pharmacother.* 1993;27:215-23.

16. Lipowski EE. Evaluating the outcomes of pharmaceutical care. *J Am Pharm Assoc.* 1996;NS36:726-34.

17. Lohr KN. Outcomes measurement: concepts and questions. *Inquiry.* 1988;25:37-50.

18. Kozma CM, Reeder CE, Schulz RM. Economic, clinical and humanistic outcomes: a planning tool for pharmacoeconomic research. *Clin Ther.* 1993;15:1121-32.

19. Angaran DM. Selecting, developing and evaluating indicators. *Am J Hosp Pharm.* 1991;48:1931-37.

20. U.S. Navy Total Quality Leadership Office. *Handbook for Basic Process Improvement.* Washington, DC: Department of Defense; 1996.

21. National Committee for Quality Assurance. State of Health Care Quality, 2003. Available at: http://www.ncqa.org/. Accessed October 16, 2003.

22. Peeples M, Mulcahy K, Tomky D, et al. The conceptual framework of the National Diabetes Education Outcomes System (NDEOS). *Diabetes Educ.* 2001;27:547-62.

23. Park JY, Daly JM. Evaluation of diabetes management software. *Diabetes Educ.* 2003;29:255-62, 267.

24. Mapi Research Institute. Quality of Life Instruments Database (QOLID). Available at: http://www.qolid.org. Accessed October 16, 2003.

25. Luscombe FA. Health-Related Quality of Life Measurement in Type 2 Diabetes. *Value Health.* 2000;3(Suppl 1):S15-28.

26. Schommer JC, Kucukarslan SN. Measuring patient satisfaction with pharmaceutical services. *Am J Health Syst Pharm.* 1997;54:2721-32.

27. Shibley MCH, Cary CH, Herbert DA. Patients' opinions about a community pharmacy diabetes care program. *J Am Pharm Assoc.* 1999;39:724-5.

Chapter 4

ACHIEVING AN ADA-RECOGNIZED-PRACTICE

Magaly Rodriguez de Bittner

IN THIS CHAPTER:

- Overview of the ADA Recognition Process
- Standard One: Organizational Structure
- Standard Two: Population and Resources
- Standard Three: Governing Body
- Standard Four: Coordinator Qualifications
- Standard Five: Instructional Team
- Standard Six: Continuing Education
- Standard Seven: Curriculum
- Standard Eight: Patient Education Plans
- Standard Nine: Documentation System
- Standard Ten: Continuous Quality Improvement
- Application Process for ADA Recognition

Background

The American Diabetes Association (ADA) has been recognizing programs in the area of diabetes education for several years. In the past, programs seeking recognition were mostly based in hospital or outpatient clinics in a variety of health care systems. It was not until the year 2000 that pharmacy-based programs started to seek ADA Recognition.

The first recognized diabetes program located in a chain pharmacy was the *Giant Pharmacy Diabetes Care Outpatient Education Program*. This program was developed as a partnership between the University of Maryland School of Pharmacy and Giant Pharmacy, and combines pharmaceutical care services, comprehensive diabetes education, and nutritional services. It is a comprehensive interdisciplinary program offered at a convenient supermarket pharmacy.

Currently there are at least 11 pharmacy-based programs around the country that have gained ADA recognition. These programs are located at pharmacy chains, independent pharmacies, and physician-group practice sites.

ADA recognition gives the diabetes education programs structure and process, providing an appropriate organizational framework as well as quality of services. It means that the education program meets the National Standards for Diabetes Self-Management Education. The ADA recognition is important because it is a symbol of quality recognized by the health care system, insurers, and patients and also insures that the organization commits resources to the education program. Programs that are recognized also have an effective organizational structure, a structured evaluation system, assessment of behavioral and clinical outcomes, and most importantly the ability to bill Medicare for diabetes education services.

In 1998, the Medicare Balanced Budget Act of 1997 was expanded to include payment for outpatient diabetes self-management training services provided by certified providers. Glucose monitors, test strips, and other monitoring supplies were also covered. Final regulations were established in February 2001. Under these regulations, a diabetes education program that has ADA recognition is eligible to apply for a Medicare provider number and receive reimbursement for diabetes education services provided to Medicare recipients who are eligible. This legislation allowed many pharmacy-based diabetes education programs to gain provider status.

ADA Recognition Process

The latest *National Standards for Diabetes Self-Management Education* were developed in 2000 and published again in 2002.[1] These standards were developed by a task force composed "of individuals from all major organizations and disciplines with significant interest in the provision of quality diabetes care and self-management education." The task force critically reviewed prior standards and developed new standards based on a comprehensive evidence-based review of the literature dealing with diabetes education.

The ADA used *National Standards for Diabetes Self-Management Education* as the basis for the 6th edition application for ADA recognition. However, the 6th edition application is frequently updated, so you should check the Web-based instructions for the application and criteria for recognition immediately before submitting an application. The Web address for up-to-date information on the ADA recognition process is www. diabetes.org/professional/recognition/erp.jsp.

Standards for Diabetes Self-Management Education (DSME) Programs

STANDARD ONE: ORGANIZATIONAL STRUCTURE

This standard deals with the organizational structure of the educational program. It establishes that the DSME entity will have documentation of its organizational structure, mission statement, and goals, and will recognize and support quality DSME as an integral part of their diabetes care services.

The standard creates the need for the educational program to have the following:

- A policy and procedures manual, which contains all the policies and procedures for the program. It includes a description of the role that pharmacists and other health care providers (dietitians, nutritionist, nurses, technicians) play in the delivery of the education, as well as who reports to whom, etc.
- Job descriptions, including those for the coordinator of the program and the instructors.
- Corporate commitment and support to the program, which involves a statement indicating the commitment of the organization to diabetes education and the program. This can be a statement from the CEO of the company, or the overall mission statement of the organization if it includes aspects of patient care and particularly diabetes education services.
- Definition of relationships and roles, which could be explained as part of the job descriptions and the organizational chart of the program.
- Guidelines and protocols followed by the educational programs, which contain a description of the services and/or program and the protocols established for the education process and assessment of the patient.

Appendix B at the end of this book contains sample documents, including examples of program descriptions (Documents 1 and 2) used at two educational programs. There is also an example of a Policies and Procedures Manual (Sample Document 3). You can use these samples to help you create your own documents.

STANDARD TWO: POPULATION AND RESOURCES

The DSME entity will determine the target population, assess educational needs, and identify the resources necessary to meet the target population's requirements for self-management education. As part of this standard, it is necessary to establish a mechanism to assess the overall educational, cultural, and health needs of the patients. The program can meet this standard by conducting a variety of assessments of their patients. Initially, as part of the needs assessment, a brief analysis of the target population in the surrounding area can help to identify health-related needs. This tool should be reassessed at each annual review.

An individual needs assessment should also be conducted for each patient who enrolls in the program. The assessment findings will help in the formulation of educational and treatment plans, and will provide a guide to the types of materials that the educator may need to use (e.g., large print, documents in another language, low grade reading materials, graphs, and pictures).

Such analyses should accomplish certain tasks. Needs assessments should:

- Define the target population based on market research.
- Define the educational needs of target population (cultural needs/ethnic background of participants).
- Assess each patient's reading ability.
- Identify barriers to access for diabetes services.
- Identify educational resources to meet the patient's needs.

An example of an annual program plan (Document 4) is in Appendix B at the end of this book. Forms related to the annual program plan (Forms 14-17) are in Appendix A, as are samples of education and assessment forms (Forms 18-21).

STANDARD THREE: GOVERNING BODY

This standard calls for the formation of an established committee, governing board, or advisory body made up of professional staff and other stakeholders. This advisory board will participate annually in a planning and review process that includes data analysis and outcome measurements. The board will also address community concerns.

Different professionals involved in diabetes education, including physicians, nurses, pharmacists, exercise physiologists, dietitians, and behavioral experts should be included in the committee. Also included are staff involved in delivering diabetes education; patients currently or formerly enrolled in the program; and representatives of the community at large. You may want to approach representatives from the local ADA chapter, citizens with interest in diabetes education, or any other patient with diabetes.

The role of this advisory board/committee is to guide all aspects of the diabetes program. The advisory board approves goals and objectives for the year, as well as written curricula, educational materials, the organizational structure of the program, its marketing plan, and its annual program review.

A summary of the annual program review is used to formulate objectives for the coming year. The findings of this report may determine the need to change the educational materials, the marketing plan, the budget, or the hours of operation. Copies of all the meeting minutes must be kept on file to satisfy this standard.

STANDARD FOUR: COORDINATOR QUALIFICATIONS

This standard defines the qualifications of the coordinator of the program. It establishes that the DSME coordinator must have academic and/or experiential preparation in program management and the care of individuals with chronic diseases. This standard does not stipulate that the coordinator must be a Certified Diabetes Educator (CDE), but the coordinator must have the educational training and experience to coordinate a diabetes education program and have completed the required number of continuing education (CE) credits in diabetes and diabetes related topics.

A pharmacist can qualify for this position if, in addition to the education received in pharmacy school, he or she has training in diabetes management and care. Such training might include a certificate program, Certified Disease Manager designation from the National Institute for Standards in Pharmacist Credentialing, or a diabetes program (consisting of more than 16 hours). Pharmacists must also earn required CE credits every year.

The coordinator will oversee the planning, implementation, and evaluation of the DSME. He or she must make sure that there is a systematic process to deliver education with the appropriate evaluation of outcomes. The coordinator is responsible for the accountability and continuity of the educational process and will oversee the DSME operations with on-site supervision. In programs using more than one site, the coordinator must conduct frequent visits to all the sites and he or she is the ultimate person responsible for their operation. At each site a manager should respond to the coordinator and keep him or her informed about management issues related to the site.

A sample job description of a coordinator is outlined in the box in the next column.

Sample Job Description of DSME Coordinator

The coordinator of the Caring Pharmacy Diabetes Care Program is a registered pharmacist with a Doctor of Pharmacy degree. She also has a strong background in diabetes education and is a Certified Diabetes Educator (certification by the National Certification Board for Diabetes Educators). The program coordinator reports to the Manager of Pharmacy Services.

Her responsibilities include:

- Serve as a liaison for the program staff, advisory committee, and administration.
- Provide and/or coordinate the orientation and continuing education for the program personnel.
- Coordinate the planning and review of the program each year.
- Participate in the evaluation of content, teaching methods, and performance of all instructors and resource personnel.
- Participate in the preparation of the program budget.
- Participate in the evaluation of the program's effectiveness.
- Serve as the chair of the advisory committee and attend all of the meetings.
- Provide assessment, teaching, and follow-up instruction to program participants as needed.
- Oversee the program with monthly on-site supervision of the diabetes care program.

STANDARD FIVE: INSTRUCTIONAL TEAM

This standard defines the type of instructors needed for the program and their profession and training. The "instructional team" is responsible for all educational content of the program. More than one instructor and more than one health profession have to be included in the team (which may include a behaviorist, exercise physiologist, pharmacist, optometrist, ophthalmologist, physician, podiatrist, registered dietitian, or registered nurse). The instructional team must consist of at least a registered dietitian and a registered nurse. On the application for ADA recognition, the instructional team should only include persons from a health profession that is eligible to sit for the CDE exam. This does not preclude others from assisting with a particular session, but the instructional team listed on the application for ADA recognition should include only health professionals.

The requirement to include a nurse and dietitian was added in the recent revision of the standards. The committee noted that most of the evidence-based data demonstrating that patients benefited from diabetes education involved teams including both a dietitian and a nurse. (Emerging data and published studies show pharmacists to be essential to the success of the team, but this data was limited at the time of the review for the new standards.) The committee stated that additional research is needed to classify other members of the team as essential. Therefore this standard does not prohibit or discourage the addition of other professionals to the team, but also does not require it.

The standard also states that the instructional staff must be CDEs or have recent didactic and experiential preparation in education and diabetes management. Primary instructors require specialized diabetes and educational training beyond their basic academic preparation. Obtaining a CDE credential is one way to demonstrate this specialized training. If the instructors are not CDEs they must demonstrate that they have adequate training prior to and during their participation in the program. Standard Six outlines the specific requirements for CE credits.

It is also important that primary instructors are given adequate time to provide education and document their services. Instructors may participate in the preparation of the annual summary and serve as members of the advisory board.

STANDARD SIX: CONTINUING EDUCATION

This standard specifies the number of hours and content of continuing education DSME instructors must have. Instructors obtain continuing education in the areas of diabetes management, behavioral interventions, teaching and learning skills, and counseling skills. In addition, the instructors must remain current in therapeutic modalities and medical nutrition therapy, as well as update their teaching skills and behavioral intervention techniques regularly.

If the instructors are not CDEs they must have at least 16 hours of DSME experience per month within 12 months of the start of the data period. They must also have completed 7.5 hours of continuing education in diabetes-related topics within the past 12 months (3 contact hours in diabetes specific topics, 3 contact hours in behavioral and learning topics, and 1.5 hours in diabetes-related topics).

If the instructor has not averaged at least 16 hours per month of DSME experience within the 12 months prior to the start of the data period, then he or she must show documentation of 16 contact hours of continuing education in diabetes-related topics within the past 12 months (10 contact hours in diabetes-specific topics, 4 hours in behavioral and learning topics, and 2 contact hours in diabetes-related topics).

STANDARD SEVEN: CURRICULUM

This standard states that a written curriculum with educational outcomes shall be available and instructors will use it to deliver the educational sessions. The initial individual assessment of the patients will determine the patients' educational needs and also which content areas are delivered during the educational sessions. For example, if during the initial individual assessment the educator establishes that the patient already possesses the knowledge and the skills to test their glucose using a glucometer, then this specific area does not need to be taught again.

The educational session must incorporate the educational needs and learning style of the patient. The educator should use a variety of educational experiences to accomplish the set of outcomes established for the patient. For each content area, there should be defined learning objectives, educational outcomes, and methods for evaluating and documenting the achievement of the educational outcomes. The topics should be covered at basic, intermediate, or advanced levels according to the educational needs of the patient.

The content areas included in the written curriculum for DSME are described in the box in the next column.

You may be able to adapt or use an existing curriculum, either from another program or one already published. One example is the *Life With Diabetes* publication from the University of Michigan Diabetes Research and Training Center.[2] This publication may be ordered from the American Diabetes Association (http://store.diabetes.org/adabooks). This curriculum is accepted by the ADA as meeting all the requirements for this standard. An example of the curriculum for one educational session in the Giant Diabetes Education Program (Document 5) is included in Appendix B. This session's written curriculum was developed using the *Life with Diabetes* curriculum, but was modified to adapt to our program and the community pharmacy setting.

Content Areas for DSME

The following content areas must be included in the written curriculum for DSME:

- Describing diabetes disease process and treatment options.
- Incorporating appropriate nutritional management.
- Incorporating physical activity into lifestyle.
- Utilizing medications (if applicable) for therapeutic effectiveness.
- Monitoring blood glucose, urine ketones (when appropriate), and using the results to improve control.
- Preventing, detecting, and treating acute complications.
- Preventing, detecting, and treating chronic complications.
- Goal setting to promote health and problem solving for daily living.
- Integrating psychosocial adjustment to daily life.
- Promoting pre-conception care, management during pregnancy, and gestational diabetes management.

STANDARD EIGHT: PATIENT EDUCATION PLANS

This standard establishes the need to have an educational plan for all patients in the program. Patients should also have periodic reassessments with the program's instructor(s). The instructor must select educational materials and teaching methods related to the patient's learning needs. He or she must also be aware of learning styles as well as appropriate educational materials and interventions aimed at meeting the teaching goals.

The educational plan must be developed using the information obtained from the patient's history. Information pertaining to the patient's medical history, cultural influences, health beliefs and attitudes, prior diabetes knowledge, self-management skills and behaviors, readiness to learn, cognitive ability, physical limitations, family support, and financial status must be taken into account when developing the educational plan and provider interventions. Examples of educational plans and a content outline are presented in Appendix B as Documents 6 and 7.

STANDARD NINE: DOCUMENTATION SYSTEM

This standard establishes the need to have a documentation system to record patient-related information, educational session content and outcomes, patients' individual assessments, education plans, interventions, evaluations, and follow-up. This documentation system must be a permanent and confidential record and should be kept in a secured place under a locking system. Providers should also ensure that all storage and sharing of health information about patients be done in compliance with the confidentiality provisions of the Health Insurance Portability and Accountability Act (HIPAA).

The system must be standardized and used by all the instructors in the program to provide evidence of collaboration among instructional staff, providers, and referral sources. Maintaining this permanent record gives educators and evaluators a tool to review diabetes care quality and check adherence to practice guidelines.

There is no specific requirement that these records be computerized. The choice of using paper forms or a computer system is left to the discretion of the program coordinator and the organization. Examples of the forms can be found in Appendix A (see Forms 2-4 and 18-21).

STANDARD TEN: CONTINUOUS QUALITY IMPROVEMENT

This standard establishes the need to have a continuous quality improvement (CQI) process to evaluate the effectiveness of the education experience and to determine opportunities for improvement. There should be goals and objectives for quality improvement that are consistent with the organizational goals of the program. The standard also establishes that the CQI process must involve continuous qualitative and quantitative analysis of processes and health and satisfaction outcomes. An example of a form used in quality assurance of documentation (Form 22) can be found in Appendix A.

However, it is important to realize that filling out a form is only a part of the quality improvement process. The information gathered from the forms should be evaluated periodically to determine if improvements in the process of care are needed. In order to evaluate outcomes, data collection instruments should be administered on multiple occasions during the program (for example, a pre- and post-program diabetes knowledge quiz, or a quality of life instrument administered every 6 months). See Chapter 3 for more information on quality improvement.

Application Process for ADA Recognition

The 6th edition application and instructions for ADA Education Recognition can be accessed from the ADA Web site at www.diabetes.org/main/professional/recognition/erp.jsp. The application form and instructions can be downloaded for review and printing.

However, the 6th edition application will only be accepted online via the ADA's Web site. It is strongly recommended that you download the "Application Form Template" from the ADA Web site and complete it on paper before attempting to apply online. This step will decrease the likelihood of errors as well as decrease the time required to fill out the application online. The section titled "Frequently Asked Questions" has useful tips that help prevent mistakes.

The fee for the application is $1,050 for the first site and $100 for each additional site affiliated with a program (effective 7/1/03). This is a nonrefundable processing fee. It can be paid by check or credit card. The same application and processing fees apply to all programs, whether they are applying for the first time or reapplying for recognition.

For multisite programs that are located in different states, the coordinator is asked to fill out a request for multisites explaining why they should be considered part of the same program. It is essential to demonstrate that the coordinator has the ability to conduct frequent on-site visits to the different sites.

Before filling out the application, your education program must meet all of the criteria in the application for 6 months prior to your application date. Also, the application requires program data collected for a period of 6 months. You must have a minimum of 20 patients in your data collection period (effective 4/03). You must submit your online application to the ADA within 3 months of the end of the data period.

Copies of various documents must be sent to the ADA with applications. The documents required are described in the box in the next column.

After the application, documents, and check are submitted and reviewed, the program will receive a score of Pass or Fail. If the program passes it will receive a certificate of recognition good for 3 years. The program must submit an annual status report to the ADA.

All programs that apply for ADA education program recognition have the chance to be selected for a random paper audit. Once the application is submitted online the program may be notified about the audit and what documents must be submitted. This documentation must be submitted to the ADA office before recognition will be awarded. All programs that achieve ADA education program recognition are subject to a random on-site audit by trained auditors. This may occur any time during the 3 years

Documents for ADA Recognition Application

Copies of various documents must accompany the application. They include:

- Letter from the Chief Administrative Officer (top official of the sponsoring organization responsible for the Diabetes Education Program) verifying the application information is correct and the sponsoring organization supports the diabetes education entity. A sample letter can be found in the "Instructions" section of the Web site.
- Copies of current licenses and registrations from all instructional team members and instructional staff members. It is recommended that the licenses, CDR card for the dietitian, and CE certificates be stapled together for each person. Highlight the expiration dates on the CDE certificates and licenses or registrations.
- Copies of CDE certificates of all CDE instructional team and instructional staff members and continuing education verification for all non-CDE instructional team and instructional staff members. Also, include CE certificate and CE program description brochure with course objectives or course outline.
- One of these support documents: minutes of the annual program plan and program review meeting of the oversight/advisory committee; program coordinator's job description and curriculum vitae or résumé; or formal CQI plan.

of recognition. To refuse an on-site audit will result in immediate loss of ADA recognition. To fail an on-site audit will result in loss of ADA recognition.

Tips for Gaining Recognition

Gaining ADA recognition for your diabetes program should be considered one of the goals for your educational program. This process can be very time-consuming and rigorous, but it provides an excellent opportunity to develop and maintain quality in your program.

ADA requirements provide a structure to follow when developing and implementing your program. Applying for recognition may help support your requests to administration for training, equipment, and documentation systems. To gain ADA recognition, these things are necessary.

Learn from other programs that have successfully obtained ADA recognition. Many program coordinators are willing to share their experiences to help you improve your program. An additional resource is a CD-ROM entitled "Diabetes Education & Recognition Resource" which can be ordered through the American Diabetes Association Web site (http:/store.diabetes.org/adabooks). The staff at the ADA Education Recognition Program is very helpful and willing to answer any questions that you may have.

You may encounter many obstacles along the way to establishing an ADA-recognized program. Don't be afraid to ask for advice or develop creative ways around the barriers. Keep your sights on your goals and try to keep everyone energized while working towards these goals. Your patients will truly appreciate your efforts to make their lives better.

References

1. American Diabetes Association. National standards for diabetes self-management education. *Diabetes Care.* 2002;25:S140-7.

2. Funnel MM, Arnold MS, Barr PA, eds. *Life with Diabetes: A Series of Teaching Outlines.* 2nd ed. Alexandria, VA: American Diabetes Association; 1997.

Appendix A
SAMPLE FORMS

Form 1

Sample Patient Consent Form

Consent for Release of Medical Information

Pharmacy Name: ____________________________________

Pharmacy Address: __________________________________

I understand that the pharmacist may need to discuss my care with my physician and other health care providers, as well as with my insurance company if required to obtain reimbursement. I do hereby grant permission for the above named pharmacy to request certain medical/health information from other members of my health care team. This information will be shared with my pharmacist confidentially and specifically for my care.

By signing my name below, I acknowledge receiving a copy of this document and agree to the sharing of my health information between the pharmacist and other members of my health care team. I understand that I may revoke this consent at any time by providing written notice to the above named pharmacy. I also understand that any release of medical information prior to my revocation shall not constitute a breach of my rights to confidentiality.

______________________	______________________
Date	Print Patient Name
______________________	______________________
Patient/Caregiver Signature	Patient Date of Birth
______________________	______________________
Relationship of Caregiver to Patient	Address
______________________	______________________
Pharmacy Representative	City, State, Zip Code

Form 2

Initial Assessment & Checklist

To be used as a tool for initially assessing a patient's needs and goals and to establish a time frame for completing the requirements of the diabetes education program. This session should not be used for detailed education; only for basic survival skills, if necessary.

Patient: ______________________________

DOB: ____________________ Date: ____________________

☐ Ukrop's Associate ☐ Study 3A Patient ☐ Richfood Employee ☐ UHC member ☐ Non-study patient

Prior to Patient Visit

- ☐ Obtain referral from physician
- ☐ Review medical history form
- ☐ Develop intervention list from medical history form and record on routine assessment form
- ☐ Determine need for initial lab-work
  - ☐ Needed ☐ Not needed
- ☐ Patient is currently on an ACE inhibitor
- ☐ Calculate BMI from med history form: ________
  BMI=kg/m^2 25-29.9=overweight >30=obesity
- ☐ Review Cardiovascular Risk Assessment
- ☐ Record present information in Tiara

Cardiovascular Risk Assessment

Y	N	
☐	☐	Diabetes
☐	☐	Patient currently smoking
☐	☐	Hypertension (BP >=140/90 or on antihypertensive med
☐	☐	HDL <40mg/dL (HDL over 60mg/dL counts as –1)
☐	☐	Male over age of 45
☐	☐	Female over age of 55
☐	☐	Family History*

_____ATPIII Relative 10-Year Risk

☐ ☐ Patient on antiplatelet/anticoagulant ________________
(Specify which agent)

During Patient Visit

(Record visit information on a routine assessment form)

- ☐ Administer Knowledge Questionnaire
- ☐ Perform labwork and vitals if needed
  - ☐ HbA1c ☐ Lipid Profile ☐ BP ☐ Pulse ☐ Weight
- ☐ Perform initial foot screening if appropriate
- ☐ Decide which classes patient will attend
- ☐ Discuss any goals that the patient would like to accomplish
- ☐ Go over survival skills if necessary for newly diagnosed patient
- ☐ Fill in Monitoring Flow Sheet
- ☐ Assess any special considerations described at right
- ☐ Fill out and give patient a Ukrop's Personal Diabetes Care Card
- ☐ Have patient sign patient contact form
- ☐ Schedule follow-up appt. for 1-2 months if appropriate

Class List

(Mark each class patient will be attending)

	Class			
☐	Why pay attention to diabetes?	Sat.	Weekday	
☐	Eating Healthy with Diabetes	Sat.	Weekday	
☐	Sunny Store Tour	Mon.	Tues.	Thurs.
☐	Medications to keep you healthy	Sat.	Weekday	
☐	Monitoring your diabetes: Not just pricking your finger	Sat.	Weekday	
☐	Increase exercise and reduce stress: Two challenging but crucial goals	Sat.	Weekday	
☐	Putting it all in perspective: How to maintain that diabetes edge	Sat.	Weekday	

Specific Patient Goals

1. ______________________________
2. ______________________________
3. ______________________________
4. ______________________________
5. ______________________________

Special Considerations

Please record any special considerations such as cultural influences, health beliefs and attitudes, readiness to learn, cognitive ability, physical limitations, family support or financial status.

____

____

____

Post Visit

- ☐ Score Knowledge Questionnaire and QOL survey
- ☐ Determine ATPIII Relative Risk and print result/include in chart
- ☐ Send a copy of this form when completed to physician along with intro letter, a copy of consent forms, a referral form to be completed, and a copy of the patient contract
- ☐ Record assessment information in Tiara
- ☐ Add patient to class roster for each class
- ☐ Fax this form to #435 (888-123-4567)

*Family history is positive if CVD or sudden death occurred in first-degree male relatives before age 55 or first-degree female relatives before age 65.

Form 3, Page 1

History of Diabetes Initial Patient Assessment

Patient Name:____
Physician:____

History of Diabetes:

Type of diabetes: ☐ Type 1 ☐ Type 2	Age when diagnosed: (age/year) __________
Family history of diabetes (*Who/type/age at dx/treatment/outcome*)	Family members who assist with diabetes management (*Name/age)*
Hospitalization(s) or ER visits for treatment of diabetes in the last 12 months (*Dates/reasons/duration/outcome)*	Physician office visits for diabetes for the last 12 months (*Date/reason/outcome*)

Diabetes Education:

Any previous diabetes education? ☐ NO ☐ YES (*When)*__________ (*Where)*__________	
What can you tell me about diabetes?	What are the symptoms of diabetes?
What is the most difficult part of having diabetes?	Do you believe your family members understand the conditions of your diabetes? ☐ YES ☐ NO (*why not?)*
Do you belong to any diabetes associations or support groups? ☐ NO ☐ YES (*organizations)*	

Form 3, Page 2

Diet/Nutrition:

Is patient under or over weight ☐Under ☐Over	Current weight:	IBW: BMI:
Any recent weight changes? (Describe)	Any recent changes in your appetite? (Describe)	
What special diet plan do you follow?	Other diet plans previously followed (*Plan/Reason for termination)*	
Have you met with a dietitian to discuss a diet plan? ☐NO ☐YES Dietitian/phone:______________________________		
What do your daily meals consist of?	When do you eat your meals?	

Exercise Plan:

Tell me about your daily activities	Do you have a regular exercise schedule? ☐ NO ☐ YES (*Type and Frequency)*
Are you exercising more or less? ☐MORE ☐LESS (*Why?)*	What things keep you from exercising?

Lab Values:

LAB VALUE	DATE/TIME	RESULT	PATIENT INTERPRETATION OF RESULTS:
Glucose			
Pharmacy Baseline Blood Glucose			
HbA1c			
TC			
LDL			
HDL			
TG			
Microalbumin/Urine Test			

Form 3, Page 3

Medications:

What medications do you use to treat your diabetes?

DRUG NAME	SCHEDULE	NUMBER OF MISSED DOSES PER WEEK	PER MONTH	SIDE EFFECTS OR ADR'S
Previously used medications to treat diabetes: *(Name of medication/dosage/reason for discontinuing medication)*				

Insulin Regimens:

	BREAKFAST		LUNCH		DINNER		BEDTIME	
Time								
Insulin Type								
Dosage (units)								
Number of Missed doses								

Please demonstrate how you draw-up and mix your insulin. *(Pharmacist Assessment)*	Syringe size: Needle size: How do you dispose of used syringes?
What problems are you having with your insulin?	Describe what is meant by rotating sites?
How do you store your insulin?	How do you carry your insulin?

Blood Glucose Monitoring:

How do you check your blood glucose levels? Does not test Visual *(test name)*________________ Urine test *(test name)* ______________ Blood Glucose Monitor *(meter name)*:______________________	How often do you monitor your blood sugars? *(Tests per day)*
What do you like about it? What do you dislike about it? Problems/difficulties you are having with the meter *(Describe)*	Please demonstrate your blood glucose monitoring technique. *(Pharmacist assessment)*
Based on the results you get from your meter, what do you consider to be high, normal, and low sugar values?	HIGH:_______ NORMAL:_______ LOW:_______

Form 3, Page 4

Hypoglycemia Awareness:

Have you ever experienced low blood sugars? ☐ NO ☐ YES *(date of last episode)*:___________ *(How often does this occur?)*:___________	Which of these symptoms have you experienced? ☐ Shakiness/trembling ☐ Tiredness ☐ Confusion/Disorientation ☐ Hunger ☐ Irritability ☐ Sweating ☐ Increase heart rate ☐ Faintness or fainted ☐ Nausea/vomiting ☐ Drowsiness/weakness
How do you treat this?	Please demonstrate your glucagon administration technique. *(Pharmacist Assessment)*

Self Care:

Foot Care	
Why is it important to check your feet on a regular basis?	How often do you inspect your feet?
What type of care do you do for your feet? ☐ Moisturize ☐ Keep toe nails trim ☐ Clean and dry feet ☐ Daily inspection ☐ Always wear shoes, no bare feet	What problems are you having with your feet?
Do you see a podiatrist for foot care? ☐ NO ☐ YES (Doctor's name/phone):______________________	
Pharmacist foot assessment	

Eye Care	
Why is it important to have your eyes examined on a yearly basis?	Date of last eye exam: Ophthalmologist name/phone:
What problems are you having with your vision?	Any problems with the following in your vision ☐ Spots ☐ Patches ☐ Areas of no vision ☐ Blurry vision ☐ Other (Describe)

Dental Care	
Why is it important to take care of your teeth and gums?	Last dentist visit: ______________________________ Dentist name/number: ___________________________
What problems are you having with your teeth or gums?	

Form 3, Page 5

Neuropathies:

Gastric Neuropathies:	☐ Difficulty Swallowing ☐ Diarrhea ☐ Nausea ☐ Anorexia	*How often, comments*
Genitourinary Tract:	☐ Dribbling ☐ Overflow Incontinence ☐ Impotence ☐ Vaginal Dryness	*How often, comments*
Cardiovascular:	☐ Orthostatic Hypotension (light headedness, pain in the neck, or visual changes) ☐ Loss of Consciousness	*How often, comments*
Regulatory System:	☐ Profuse Sweating ☐ Heat Intolerance	*How often, comments*
Peripheral Neuropathies:	☐ Decreased Heat and Light Touch Sensation ☐ Burning ☐ Tingling ☐ Numbness ☐ Intense Pain ☐ Diminished Sense of Touch, Vibration, and Temperature	*How often, comments*

Sick Day Care:

How do you take care of your diabetes when you are ill?	How often do you miss doses of your medication while you are sick?
How often do you monitor your blood sugar when you are ill?	How often do you check your urine for ketones?

Pharmacist Assessment: ______________________________

____

____

____

Plan: ______________________________

____

____

____

Pharmacist's signature:______________________________

Date:______________________

Form 4, Page 1

Routine Assessment Form

To be used at each wellness center visit to document the patient interaction and follow the patient's progress toward established goals.

Patient Name: ______________________________ DATE: ____________

Health Care Provider visits since last assessment:
Provider: __________ Last Visit: __________ Last Wellness Center Visit: __________
Provider: __________ Last Visit: __________
Subjective:
Current Complaints: ______________________________
____
Any change in medications? IF Yes explain ______________________________
Since the last Wellness Center Visit:
ER visits _____ Hospitalizations _____ Unscheduled MD Visits _____ Work Days Missed _____
Explanation: ______________________________
HMBG - Avg. readings per day over the last 2 weeks _____

Symptoms of low blood sugar

☐Shaky ☐Rapid Heart beat ☐Sweating
☐Headache ☐Hunger ☐Nausea
☐Confused ☐Other ☐NONE

Symptoms of high blood sugar

☐Dry, itchy skin ☐ ↑Thirst ☐ ↑Hunger
☐Frequent infections ☐Nocturia ☐ ↑Urination
☐Slow healing cuts ☐Fatigue ☐Blurred vision
☐Sudden weight loss ☐Other ☐NONE

Explanation

____
____
____
____
____
____

Diet Self-Assessment
Patient's self assessment of compliance with diet: ☐Good ☐Fair ☐Poor
____
____

Exercise ______________________________
____
____

Nutrition ______________________________
____
____

Monitoring ______________________________
____
____

Medications ______________________________
____
____

Form 4, Page 2

Objective

Present Time ___________ Time of last meal ___________

Blood Glucose today ___________mg/dL ☐Random ☐Fasting ☐2hr PP HbA1c _____%

Blood Pressure today _____/_____mmHg _____/_____mmHg ☐LA ☐RA ☐Sitting ☐Standing

Pulse today _____bpm. ☐Reg ☐Irreg. Weight ___________lbs

TC ___________mg/dL HDL ___________mg/dL TRG ___________mg/dL LDL ___________mg/dL

Foot inspection performed? ☐yes ☐no (See foot care form for results)

Classes patient has attended since last assessment:

☐ Why Pay Attention to Diabetes
☐ Medications to Keep You Healthy
☐ Increase Exercise and Reduce Stress
☐ Eating Healthy with Diabetes
☐ Monitoring Your Diabetes
☐ Putting It All in Perspective
☐ Sunny Store Tour

Assessment/Plan

____

____

____

____

____

____

____

____

____

____

Progress toward goals:

1. ______________________________
2. ______________________________
3. ______________________________
4. ______________________________

Issues to discuss with physician:

____

____

Results: ______________________________

Focus of next visit:

____

____

Appt. Date & Time: ___________________

Provider Signature: ______________________ Date: ___________

Source: Reprinted with permission from Ukrop's Pharmacy.

Form 5

Sample Letter to Physician

Date

Dear Dr. Smith,

I would like to take this opportunity to introduce myself and the new **Ukrop's Pharmacy Diabetes Education and Management Program**. My name is **Sarah Pharmacist** and I am a staff pharmacist at the Ukrop's Pharmacy at Virginia Center Marketplace. Ukrop's, in collaboration with **Hanover Family Physicians** and the **VCU School of Pharmacy**, has developed a comprehensive diabetes program to be offered at five of our pharmacies. I am including information on our program and hope you will find it a more convenient alternative to some of the diabetes programs already available in this area.

One of your patients, **John Doe** DOB 07/30/1937, is interested in participating in this program. To my knowledge, **Mr. Doe** has not participated in an education program previously. We have already signed him up for a few classes and would like to obtain a referral from you for this service. Please take a moment to fill in the necessary laboratory information and fax this form back to us at your earliest convenience. This form may also be used to indicate any specific goals that you may have for this patient.

Thank you for taking the time to read over the enclosed information. I look forward to working with you to help educate your patients with diabetes. Please call me if you have any questions at all and I look forward to meeting you in the near future.

Many Thanks,

Sarah Pharmacist, RPh, CDE

Source: Reprinted with permission from Ukrop's Pharmacy.

Form 6

Diabetes Screening Results

Diabetes is a disease in which the body cannot use sugar (also referred to as glucose) properly. About **17 million** people in the United States have diabetes. Approximately 1/3 of these have not been diagnosed. This means that they do not know they have diabetes. It is important to diagnose diabetes early to limit the complications that occur over time. These long-term complications include damage to the eyes, kidneys, heart, nerves, and blood vessels in the legs, feet, and hands.

Pre-diabetes is a condition somewhere between "normal" and diabetes. Because pre-diabetes often leads to diabetes, it must be diagnosed to help prevent or delay the start of diabetes itself.

Your chances of developing type 2 diabetes (the more common form) are greater if you:

- Are over age 45
- Have a family history of diabetes
- Have low HDL cholesterol or high triglycerides
- Belong to certain racial and ethnic groups (e.g., African Americans, Latinos, Asian & Pacific Islanders, and Native Americans)
- Are a woman who had gestational diabetes, a form of diabetes occurring in 2% to 5% of all pregnancies, or who has had a baby weighing 9 pounds or more at birth
- Are overweight
- Do not exercise regularly

Many symptoms can occur if a patient has diabetes. Each patient will have different symptoms. Some patients have severe symptoms while others have no symptoms at all.
Some symptoms of diabetes include:

- Frequent urination
- Unusual thirst
- Unusual weight loss
- Extreme fatigue
- Irritability
- Cuts/bruises that are slow to heal
- Frequent infections
- Blurred vision
- Extreme hunger
- Tingling/numbness in the hands or feet
- Recurring skin, gum, or bladder
- infections

To get a truly accurate screening test, the patient should be tested fasting (after having not eaten for 8 hours) or 2 hours after an oral glucose challenge (Oral Glucose Tolerance Test or OGTT), which mimics a meal. If neither of these apply, this test may not be accurate. In addition, this is only a screening test and should not be considered a diagnosis of any condition.

Normal	Fasting	After Meal or OGTT
	<110mg/dL	<140mg/dL

Date:________________

_____________mg/dL

Time:________________ Date and Time last food or beverage consumed:______________

Source: Website of the American Diabetes Association: www.diabetes.org.

Form 7

Physician Referral Form

Please fax this form to the number listed below and keep in the patient chart.

Patient Name: ______________________ Home Phone: ______________
SSN: ______________ DOB: __________ Work Phone: ______________
Insurance Company: ______________ ID#: __________ Auth#: __________
Specific Patient Needs or Impairments: ______________________________
____

Desired Services: ***You may leave this up to us or the patient by leaving the following block blank.***

Complete "Living Healthy With Diabetes" Multidisciplinary ***ADA Recognized*** Education Program ($XXX)

Group Classes from "Living Healthy With Diabetes" Offered Separately ($XX or $XX)

☐ Why Pay Attention to Diabetes? ($XX)
☐ Medications to Keep You Healthy ($XX)
☐ Putting It All In Perspective ($XX)
☐ Eating Healthy with Diabetes and the Sunny Store Tour ($XX)
☐ Monitoring Your Diabetes: Not Just Pricking Your Finger ($XX)
☐ Increase Exercise and Reduce Stress: Two Challenging But Crucial Goals ($XX)

Pharmacist Services –Individual Education Modules (15-20 min. each) - $XX

☐ Diabetes Overview
☐ Developing an effective activity program
☐ Foot care at home, work, and play
☐ Behavior change strategies and goal setting with diabetes
☐ Master your monitor
☐ Mastering your insulin therapy
☐ Sick day management
☐ Self-care and avoiding complications
☐ Stress and its effects on blood sugar
☐ Medication review and management strategies

Dietitian Services (Conducted by a Registered Dietitian)
Individual nutrition counseling specific to diabetes - $XX/hr

Diagnosis:	Complications:	Other Medical Conditions:	Other:
☐ Type 1	☐ Neuropathy	☐ Hypertension	__________
☐ Type 2	☐ Nephropathy	☐ Hypercholesterolemia	__________
☐ Gestational	☐ Retinopathy	☐ Congestive Heart Failure	__________
☐ Other __________	☐ CV Disease	☐ Overweight/Obesity	

	Value	Date		Value	Date
HbA1c	______%	________	HDL	______mg/dL	________
Total Cholesterol	______mg/dL	________	LDL	______mg/dL	________
			Triglycerides	______mg/dL	________

For the complete program, a Ukrop's dietitian will determine an appropriate calorie level for the patient and recommend an exercise program and daily aspirin therapy, unless an exception is noted below.
These ADA guidelines will be followed unless an exception is noted below: **(plasma values)**

Goals of therapy: **HbA1c< 7%** **LDL< 100mg/dL** **Fasting BS 90-130mg/dL** **Bedtime BS 110-150mg/dL**

☐ Exception______________________________________

I am referring the above-mentioned patient to the diabetes education and management program at Ukrop's Pharmacy. I believe this is a necessary part of this patient's diabetes treatment.

Physician Signature: ______________________ Date: __________ Phone: __________

FAX TO 800-123-4567

Source: Reprinted with permission from Ukrop's Pharmacy.

Form 8

Diabetes Care Services Local Needs Assessment

Patient Population	
What is the estimated diabetes population in your community? (*Nationally, 7.3% of the population is diagnosed)*	
What is the demographic breakdown of the population in your community? (*Age, race, education)*	
Access to Diabetes Education	
Are there providers of diabetes education within your community? (Independent Centers, CDEs, hospitals, etc.)	
What diabetes care services do these providers offer? *(Disease education, lifestyle education, diabetes management, diet/nutrition, medication management, monitoring)*	
Where is diabetes education offered? *(physician offices, assisted living facilities, community pharmacies, libraries, etc.)*	
Are there geographic areas within the community that lack diabetes care services?	
Practice Site Needs Assessment	
Do you currently have direct access to patients with diabetes? *(Retail pharmacy practice, physician relationships, etc.)*	
Are there large physician practices in your area to provide you with patient referrals?	
Do you have dedicated office space to deliver diabetes care services? *(Space within a pharmacy, physician practice, outpatient center)*	
Do you have the clinical tools to optimally educate and monitor patient outcomes? *(Access to HbA1c results, blood glucose monitors, CLIA waivers, biohazard procedures, computer access, etc.)*	
Payers	
What do the existing diabetes programs charge for services? *(Hourly rate, flat fee, membership)*	
Do patients pay out-of-pocket for diabetes care services?	
Who are the large employers within your community?	
Are any of these employers self-insured?	
Are any of the large physician practices in your community heavily capitated?	
Do you have access to county or city risk managers or human resource officers?	
Do you have access to health maintenance organization (HMO) or managed care organization (MCO) case managers, disease management departments, or marketing managers?	

Form 9

Action Planning Timeline and Responsibilities Chart

Action Steps to Implement Diabetes Patient Care Services	Person Responsible	Target Date
Establish a network of diabetes care pharmacists, including training, consultation areas, administration		
Develop collaborative relationships with physicians to support the program and care model		
Identify and market diabetes care services to local self-insured providers and obtain commitment for payment		
Adopt standardized care processes and outcome monitoring measures		
Develop a payment schedule and processes for payment for services		
Work with the employer(s) to establish processes for enrolling employees and tracking economic outcomes		

Form 10

Administrative Budget

Background Information:

The Administrative Budget defines the direct "out-of-pocket" costs associated with developing a pharmaceutical care practice. Not every item included in the spreadsheet will pertain to all practice settings. In these instances, please leave the particular line item blank when calculating the working budget. The total administrative budget will serve as the breakeven point when determining practice-site profitability and patient-load goals.

Administrator/Manager (pharmaceutical care practice may not have a separate site manager)

Salary	$ 65,000.00
Benefits	$ 15,000.00
Payroll Taxes	$ 5,000.00
Travel	$ 5,000.00
	$ 90,000.00

Clinical Coordinator (pharmacists responsible for patient-related activities)

Salary	$ 30,000.00
Benefits	$ 5,000.00
Payroll Taxes	$ 2,500.00
Travel	
Number of Clinicians	1
	$ 37,500.00

Administrative Staff (site may utilize office assistants, pharmacy technicians or outside office support)

Wages	$ 5,000.00
Benefits	$ 1,000.00
Payroll Taxes	$ 1,000.00
	$ 7,000.00

General and Administrative Expenses

Rent	$ 10,000.00
Utilities	$ 500.00
Telephone	$ 500.00
Equipment Lease	
Office Supplies	
Clinical Supplies	
Postage	
Advertising	
Bank Charges	
Insurance	
Legal/Accounting	
Training/Continuing Educat ion	
Software/Data Collection	
	$ 11,000.00

Total Practice Expenses	$145,500.00

Form 11

Operational Projections

Interventions Per Day

Hours Available Per Day	8
Minutes Per Intervention	30
Documentation/Follow Up (Hours)	1.5
Lunch (Minutes)	30
Maximum Visits Per Day	**12**

Practice Revenues

Break-even Revenue Per Claim *(calculated on the Break-even Analysis form)*	Per Claim Revenue can be determined either by a flat fee per intervention or by an hourly rate	$ 50.52
Projected Revenue Per Claim		$ 100.00
Number of Claims Per Day	Calculated above as "Maximum Visits Per Day"	12
Office Days Per Week		5
Office Weeks Per Year	Vacation, sick time and training must be accounted for when accurately determining practice goals	48
Total Expected Revenue		**$288,000.00**

Practice Site Projected Profits

Total Expected Revenue	$288,000.00
Total Practice Expenses	$145,500.00
Projected Profits	**$142,500.00**

Weekly Hours Commitment

Expected Patient Case Load		125
Minutes Per Intervention	Carried down from above information	30
Documentation/Follow Up/Patient (Minutes)	Calculated from above entry "Documentation/Follow up (hours)"	8
Average Visits Per Patient Per Month		1
Monthly Dedicated Patient Hours		**78**
Weekly Dedicated Patient Hours		**20**

Form 12

Break-even Analysis

Patient Load

Administrative Budget		$145,500.00
Revenue Per Claim		$ 50.52
Average Visit Per Patient	Estimated total number of visits per patient	6
Annual Revenue Per Patient		$ 303.13
Target Patient Population		**480**

Reimbursement Per Intervention

Administrative Budget	$145,500.00
Total Intervention Per Year	2880
Minimum Reimbursement Per Claim	**$ 50.52**

Form 13

Quality Improvement Team Statement

Process Definition	
Name of Process	
Boundaries of Process	
Process Improvement Objective	
Team Leadership and Members	
Team Leader	
Team Members	
Team Definitions	
Begin Date	
End Date	
Meeting Frequency	
Decision-Making Authority	
Resources Available	
Reporting Requirements	
Other Information	

Management's Signature: ______________________________ Date: __________________

Source: Navy Total Quality Leadership Office. *Handbook for Basic Process Improvement* [adaptation]. Washington, DC: Department of Defense;1996:5:1-40.

Form 14

Diabetes Wellness Program Service Area Evaluation and Checklist

Purpose:
The service area of a diabetes self-management education program must be outlined. This checklist will assist the clinician in identifying where the Diabetes Wellness Program can draw its participants.

Pharmacy Site (Address, description of pharmacy layout)
Pharmacist(s) *Diabetes Education and Clinical Training Completed*
Reference Points (Service Area) *Zip Codes/County Borders*
Estimate of General Population
Target Population Estimates
Transportation Access

Medical Care facilities in the service area defined			
Hospitals	County Health Departments	Primary Care Physicians	ADA-recognized Diabetes Programs

Form 15

Sample Annual Program Plan Two

Annual Review and Program Plan (Program # 2)
08/16/03

This is the yearly evaluation by the advisory system of DSME operations and performance as well as the program plan for the coming year based on the findings of the annual review.

1. **Goal achievement:** Review status of goals and/or objectives established for the program.

   Review: Goals/objectives for 2003 are included, as are goals/objectives for the coming year.
   Plan: Review goal achievement during the next annual review

2. **Data analysis**: Analyze and review participant access data, follow-up rates, and other relevant data.

   Review: Not able to review at this point.
   Plan: Will compile data to be reviewed at a later date.

3. **Mission statement**: Review mission statement and determine appropriateness to program operations.

   Review: Adequate.
   Plan: Review mission statement during the next annual review.

4. **Organizational structure**: Review organizational structure to assess whether the current structure is meeting the needs of the program operations and participants.

   Review: Adequate.
   Plan: Review organizational structure during the next annual review.

5. **Population served**: Analyze and review participant population data and assess how the program is meeting the needs of the population it is serving.

   Review: Adequate.
   Plan: Review population served during the next annual review.

6. **Resources**: Review adequacy of resources, including personnel, budget, equipment, and curriculum.

   Review: Adequate.
   Plan: Review adequacy of resources during the next annual review.

7. **Behavioral and other outcome data measurements of program participants**: Evaluate effectiveness of program based on behavioral goals and other outcome measurement data.

   Review: No hard data to look at; however, the program seems to be effective based on participant and instructor feedback.
   Plan: Review during the next annual review.

Form 16

Goals/Objectives

2003

- Develop and begin to provide diabetes patient education classes in July and August of 2003 in 2 Caring pharmacies.
  Status: Completed
- Investigate reimbursement opportunities for our program from area employers and insurers.
  Status: We have done some limited investigation and have been able to contract with one local insurer, Healthcare.
- Develop a policy for Caring Pharmacy's employees to receive this program at no cost to them through the health plan.
  Status: Completed
- Develop a marketing plan to expand the program to patients we may not already be marketing to.
  Status: While there is no formal marketing plan in place, a brochure has been developed and will be distributed soon. We will continue to develop our marketing strategies.
- Ensure that a process is in place to track data for ADA recognition as well as for program analysis and patient outcomes.
  Status: The software is being used to track data for ADA recognition. Currently we have no software for program analysis and patient outcomes. This is being investigated.

2004-2005

- Continue to provide a unique diabetes patient education program in 4 Caring Pharmacy locations by enrolling patients in the program at the 4 locations in September and into 2005.
- Investigate compensation opportunities for the program from area employers and insurers by meeting with employers and insurers to discuss the possibility of arranging a compensation package.
- Expand the program to patients and health care professionals who may not be aware of the program by developing a marketing plan and brochure for the program.
- Obtain recognition from the American Diabetes Association by gathering data for and submitting an application for ADA recognition.
- Investigate possible grant or research opportunities.
- Expand the program to the Heartfelt Caring Pharmacy Location in September 2004.

Annual Program Review

A. **Review of Program Objectives for the year 2003**

1. **Clinical:**

a. To reduce the individual HbA1c of program participants by 1% point in a 12-month period unless the patient is already within the target range.

Results: Objective not met. A total of 18 patients signed up for the program during the review period. A total of fourteen patients only wanted to do one or two sessions. The sessions most commonly requested by the patients were the overview (n = 6), monitoring (n = 6) and nutrition (n = 5) sessions. Four of these 18 have completed the program through follow-up. Of these we had HbA1c results in three patients preprogram. In one case, we did not get any laboratory data from the physician even after repeated attempts to get the information. Not all the patients had a hemoglobin A1c drawn post-program even after recommendations were made to the physicians. We were able to obtain pre and post HbA1c data in one patient. The mean HbA1c was reduced by approximately 2.1% postprogram. This data does not reflect a 12-month period, because all patients completed the program in less than 12 months. Due to the laboratory regulations governing the testing procedures of this test we are unable to measure HbA1c at the pharmacy. We depend on the physicians to order this test, and in some cases they are not doing so. In addition, we had a change in personnel within the program that caused disruptions in the follow-up mechanism to obtain the data.

b. To increase by 20% the percentage of participants that have an annual dilated retinal exam by increasing visits to the ophthalmologist.

Results: Objective met. A total of 18 patients signed up for the program during the review period. A total of fourteen patients only wanted to do one or two sessions. The sessions most commonly requested by the patients were the overview (n = 6), monitoring (n = 6) and nutrition (n = 5) sessions. Four of these 18 have completed the program through follow-up. All 4 patients were educated as to the importance of yearly dilated retinal eye exams. All 4 patients agreed to schedule an eye exam in the next 3 months. The results indicate that it is very difficult to assess if the patient actually had a dilated eye exam performed.

2. **Behavioral:**

a. To increase by 20% the percentage of program participants performing a daily foot exam.

Results: Objective met. All four patients who completed the program were educated about the need to perform daily foot exams and how to do so. At each subsequent visit all patients were assessed as to whether they were performing daily foot exams. All patients stated they were, bringing the percentage of program participants doing foot exams to 100%.

b. To increase by 20% the percentage of program participants that monitor blood glucose at home on a regular basis.

Form 17, Page 2

Results: Objective met. All of the four patients who completed the program were educated about the importance of blood glucose monitoring and its relationship to therapy and self-management. Each was then offered a meter and instructed on how to use it. All four chose to do so, increasing the percentage of program participants monitoring at home to 100%.

3. **Administrative**:

a. Increase the number of program participants to 30 a year per site.

Results: Objective not met. A total of 18 patients have enrolled in the program during the review period. Limited marketing as well as financial barriers for the target population may be likely reasons why this objective was not met. The fact that we do not have an agreement with insurance companies for financial compensation makes it harder to recruit the target number of patients. Since this is a new, unique, and innovative program, patients and providers need to become familiar and comfortable with these services. We are starting to see more physician referrals.

B. Comparison between target and actual audience

Target Audience: Adults patients with Type 1, Type 2 diabetes, and their families.

Actual Audience was: Based on statistics from June 2002 to December 2003, the actual audience was the same as our target audience. A large majority of patients were elderly, had type 2 diabetes, and were African-American.

Discussion: N/A

Action: N/A

C. Ease by which participants enter or access the program

Procedure for responding to requests for information and referrals: Potential patients interested in learning more about the program are given an informational pamphlet and immediately offered an appointment for a free 15-minute individual consultation to learn more about the program. Patients referred by physicians can schedule their first education session in person at the sites or by calling the site at any time during operational hours. Patients can enter the program immediately; there is no waiting period.

Discussion: Patients are easily able to schedule free consultations or educational sessions around their personal schedules. The program is offered two days a week every week during afternoon and evening hours, which allows flexibility for individual patients. They can enter the program immediately.

Action: No action is necessary at this time since the program is easily accessible to most patients.

How participants enter the program: Patients enter the program through physician, pharmacist, or self-referral.

Number of participants who entered the program this year (June 02-Dec 03): 18

Number of participants who entered the program last year: 22

Discussion: Program enrollment continues to be relatively low and has declined since its inception in November of 2001. This is not due to lack of interest from patients, as over 48 free consultations have been performed despite limited marketing. A potential reason for the decline in enrollment may be that the patients who are willing to pay cash for the services at the sites have been identified and contacted. The major barrier to enrollment based on patient feedback has been cost and lack of insurance coverage. Approximately 80% of patients choosing not to enroll stated cost as the primary reason, as well as the fact that their insurance does not cover the cost of the services.

Action: To increase enrollment, marketing strategies need to be expanded. Physician office detailing needs to take place, especially now that we have ADA recognition.

Waiting period to enter the program: There is no waiting period to enter the program at this point.

Discussion: N/A

Action: N/A

D. Participant follow-up mechanisms

The *number and percentage* of all participants who completed the program through follow-up assessment: Of the 18 patients who entered the program through the data period, 4 (22%) completed all eight educational sessions and one follow-up session.

Discussion: Follow-up rates have been variable. Some patients signed for only one or two sessions; other patients signed for the whole program but failed to complete all sessions (n = 3). Allowing the patients the opportunity to do four sessions instead of eight (if they wish to do so) has helped somewhat and will continue to increase the number of patients who will complete ALL sessions. Also, some type of incentive program for attending follow-up should be explored, such as a certificate of completion.

Action: Continue offering patients the opportunity to complete the program in four or eight sessions. Offering the program in four condensed sessions will allow a small decrease in the price of the program. We will continue to reassess patient acceptance of each option to determine if we should continue to offer eight sessions. Incentives to patients to complete the sessions such as a certificate of completion, will be offered. Maybe we should also consider developing a support group for patients who completed the program or offering a newsletter. The Diabetes Club that Caring Pharmacy just instituted may also be an incentive.

E. Program Resources

Personnel:

Discussion: Currently we have 1.5 FTE pharmacist educators and .25 dietitians. The current personnel are adequate to meet the needs of the program at this time. We need to start exploring whether to add a nurse to meet the new ADA Recognition requirements of having a nurse and a dietitian in the team.

Form 17, Page 4

Action: Personnel is adequate for the current demand. If there is expansion of the program, more pharmacists will need to be trained. Currently, three other pharmacists are planning to attend the Lifescan training program this year.

Space:

Discussion: Currently we have two counseling offices for individual education and follow-up sessions. We need to start developing group sessions to be able to bill Medicare. These sessions can take place in the counseling rooms (for 2-3 patients) or we may need to identify another area in the pharmacy.

Action: Explore options for space to provide the opportunity for group counseling sessions for those patients who prefer group counseling and as per Medicare requirements.

Budget:

Discussion: We need to have a budget assigned from corporate headquarters to assess financial impact of the program.

Action: To obtain a budget for each of the stores.

F. Curriculum, educational materials, and community resource list

Curriculum/Instructional Methods:

Discussion: Currently we use the Life with Diabetes curriculum; this has been an acceptable curriculum. We need to make sure that the modules are reviewed to include new diabetes drugs introduced in the market. We also need the dietitians (since we have had changes in the staff recently) to review the nutrition module and feel comfortable with the educational content of this session.

Action: We will review ALL modules to update the necessary information. Dietitians will be asked to review the nutrition module. Instructional materials and supplies for group sessions need to be obtained to accommodate this teaching method.

Educational Materials: (Answer Yes/No)

Yes **accurate** _Yes_ **current**

appropriate for target audience
Yes low literacy
Yes foreign language
Yes culturally sensitive
Yes readability
Yes age-specific
_No_ special needs

Discussion: We have obtained culturally sensitive materials and have materials written in other languages. We need to review other materials available from the AADE, National Diabetes Education Program, and ADA to see if we should also use those too.

Action: We will search for and review educational materials from AADE, NDEP, and ADA.

Form 17, Page 5

Community Resource List: (Answer Yes/No) _No_ **appropriate for target audience**

Discussion: Need to obtain community resources to include more local programs for patients.

Action: We will conduct a review of all available programs in the Love and Friendship areas and local groups to update the Resource List.

G. Marketing

How and when program is marketed to the target population: Potential patients at each site are identified upon dispensing of diabetes medications. These patients are given an informational pamphlet in their medication bag and are asked to speak with the pharmacist about the program. Pamphlets are also displayed near the pharmacy counter at each site. Nearby stores have been provided with pamphlets and are following similar methods of patient identification. One advertisement was placed in the Caring Pharmacy insert of the newspaper in the Love area. No other media advertisement has taken place.

Primary Referral Sources: Self-referral, pharmacist referral, and physician referral.

Discussion: Referrals have decreased over the past year for the reasons discussed above. All marketing materials need to be revised to reflect the fact that we are ADA recognized.

Action: Marketing materials will be revised. Physician detailing needs to take place.

H. Program effectiveness and participant outcomes

Summary of Behavioral Goals:

Number of participants who completed program: 4
Number who selected behavior to change: 4
Number lost to follow-up: 1
Evaluation Scale: _0_ = never _3_ = always

Behavior	Number of times behavior chosen	Number of times rated	% Attainment
Monitoring	1	1	100%
Nutrition	3	3	100%
Increase physical activity	1	1	100%
Foot care	4	4	100%

Form 17, Page 6

Discussion: All 4 participants who completed the program selected behaviors to change. The program has been successful at improving the selected behaviors of monitoring, foot care, increase physical activity, and nutrition. All participants are now examining their feet daily and monitoring their blood glucose at home on a regular basis and are able to demonstrate the correct technique for doing so. Four patients also selected changes in nutrition behaviors. All of these patients had sessions with a nutritionist and developed specific meal planning skills and meal plans. In some cases specific nutrition goals were not clearly stated and therefore were difficult to assess during follow-up. More attention will be paid to clearly defining goals, nutrition-related and others, and assessing and documenting each specific goal at every session and at follow-up.

Action: Instructors will be reminded to assess educational goals at each session and during the follow-up sessions.

Summary of other outcome measure:

Discussion of results: The other outcome measure selected for this year was hemoglobin A1c. Not all patients had a hemoglobin A1c drawn pre-program or post-program. In some cases, the physician did not send the information. Monitoring of HbA1c on a regular basis is not routine for the majority of the physicians. Due to the laboratory regulations governing the testing procedures of this test in Maryland, we are unable to measure HbA1c at the pharmacy. We depend on the physicians to order this test.

Action: Consider changing the outcome to assess not only impact on HbA1c but also to improve the frequency of HbA1c monitoring as recommended by the ADA by contacting the physician by phone and in writing when the tests are not being performed. Also, explore the possibility of obtaining a waiver from the Department of Health to allow us to conduct the test in the store or to use the outpatient HbA1c test, where patients can send the sample in the mail and obtain the results. Explore the possibility of using other outcomes measures such as fructosamine.

Form 18, Page 1

Diabetes Self-Management Education Record

Patient Name: ______________________________

Instructions: Please indicate teaching code, outcome code, date, and initials

Teaching Codes:
V = verbal instruction, W = written instruction, A = audio visual, D = demonstration, R = return demo

Assessment/Outcome codes:
C = competent, RA = requires assistance, N = needs review, U = unable, NA = not applicable

TOPIC ■ Objectives	Initial Assessment codes/initials/ date	Teaching Methods codes/initials/date	Outcome/ Reinforcement codes/initials/ date	Comments
DIABETES OVERVIEW				
■ Define diabetes mellitus				
■ State similarities and differences between Type 1 and Type 2 diabetes				
■ Describe reason for controlling blood glucose				
■ State desired blood glucose ranges				
■ Recognize three tests used by health care providers to monitor diabetes				
■ Identify personal goals for blood glucose control				
STRESS AND PSYCHOSOCIAL ADJUSTMENT				
■ Demonstrate skills in adjusting to living with diabetes				
■ Describe feelings about having diabetes				
■ List body changes that occur during stress				
■ Demonstrate appropriate coping management skills				
■ Identify additional support resources				
■ Set meaningful goals				
FAMILY INVOLVEMENT AND SOCIAL SUPPORT				
■ Demonstrate family understanding of diabetes				
■ Describe how family support affects blood glucose control				
NUTRITION				
■ Describe importance of meal planning				
■ Describe relationship of weight loss to diabetes control				
■ Discuss importance of meal timing, portion sizes, and food variety				
■ Determine food groups various foods belong to				

Form 18, Page 2

■ Describe diabetes nutritional guidelines				
■ Demonstrate understanding of food labels				
■ Discuss safety concerns of diabetes and alcohol				
INSULIN				
■ Describe what insulin is and how it works				
■ Name type(s) of insulin and activity profile				
■ Describe storage of insulin and quality assurance measures				
■ Describe measurement and administration				
■ Demonstrate injection administration technique				
■ Identify possible side effects				
■ Adjust dosages schedule appropriately				
■ Demonstrate proper sharps disposal				
MONITORING AND USE OF RESULTS				
■ Describe benefits of self monitoring				
■ Demonstrate accurate use of own equipment and log				
■ State target glucose range				
■ Adjust plan based on results				
■ Identify factors that may cause inaccurate readings				
■ State when, how, and why to test urine for ketones				
■ Describe actions for ketonuria				
■ Define HbA1c and target goals				
RELATIONSHIPS AMONG NUTRITION, EXERCISE, MEDICATION, AND BLOOD GLUCOSE				
■ Summarize the relationship between nutrition, exercise, medication, and blood glucose control				
EXERCISE AND ACTIVITY				
■ Describe the general benefits of exercise				
■ Explain the effect of exercise on glucose control				
■ List safe exercise activities and safety factors to consider				
■ Demonstrate measures to prevent hypoglycemic episodes				
MEDICATIONS (ORAL, ETC.)				
■ Describe how oral medications work				
■ Name medication(s) used to treat diabetes				

Form 18, Page 3

■ Explain dosage and administration schedule				
■ List potential side effects and adverse drug reactions				
■ List what to do when patient misses dose of medication(s)				
■ Describe the importance of review of over the counter medications before use				
■ Describe the effects of other medications on blood sugar				
PREVENTION, DETECTION, AND TREATMENT OF ACUTE COMPLICATIONS				
HYPOGLYCEMIA				
■ Define and list causes of hypoglycemia				
■ Describe signs and symptoms				
■ Describe and demonstrate treatment regimens				
■ Verify that family member knows when and how to use a glucagon				
■ Know when to contact medical assistance				
■ Use medical alert ID				
HYPERGLYCEMIA				
■ Define and list causes of hyperglycemia				
■ Describe signs and symptoms				
■ Make monitoring adjustments				
■ Know when to contact medical assistance				
SICK DAY MANAGEMENT				
■ List symptoms of ketoacidosis				
■ Describe sick day management plan				
■ Demonstrate ketone testing technique				
■ Identify when to contact physician				
PREVENTION, DETECTION, AND TREATMENT OF CHRONIC COMPLICATIONS				
■ Explain the relationship of blood glucose control on complications				
■ Name the chronic complications of diabetes				
■ List factors of atherosclerosis				
■ Identify signs and symptoms of neuropathy				
PERSONAL HEALTH HABITS				
FOOT CARE				
■ State reason for daily self-inspection of feet				
■ Demonstrate how to examine feet				
■ Describe signs and symptoms of potential foot problems and need for prompt medical attention				

Form 18, Page 4

■ State need for foot exam at each office visit				
SKIN CARE				
■ Describe signs and symptoms of infection				
■ Demonstrate proper skin care				
DENTAL CARE				
■ Describe proper dental care				
■ State need for regular dental exams				
BEHAVIOR CHANGE STRATEGIES, GOAL SETTING, RISK FACTOR REDUCTION				
■ List factors to control and reduce risk				
■ Discuss benefits of self-care				
■ Demonstrate ability to change for a healthier quality of life				
■ Set meaningful goals				
BENEFITS, RISKS, AND MANAGEMENT OPTIONS FOR IMPROVING GLUCOSE CONTROL				
■ List benefits of improving control and methods				
■ State role in prevention of complications				
PRECONCEPTION CARE, PREGNANCY, GESTATIONAL DIABETES				
■ Define gestational diabetes				
■ Describe the importance of blood glucose control in diabetes				
■ Identify risks of diabetes in pregnancy				
■ State goals of pregnancy care for a woman with diabetes				
■ List meal planning goals to assist in glucose control				

INITIALS	SIGNATURE

Form 19

Diabetes Wellness Program Patient Flow Chart

Patient Name: ______________________________

Instructions: Please indicate dates of exam, test, or assessment and the actual results when appropriate. Additional explanations should be written in the patient's pharmacy chart.

	Initial consult Date/result	Date/result	Date/result	Date/result
GENERAL OFFICE VISITS				
▪ Review management plan. *Type 1 every 3 months, Type 2 every 3-6 months*				
GLYCEMIC CONTROL				
▪ Review medications *(every visit)*				
▪ Review blood glucose target goal *(every visit)*				
▪ HbA1c Test *(every 3-6 months)*				
▪ Review HbA1c target goal *(every visit)*				
▪ Weight, Height, BMI				
KIDNEY FUNCTION				
▪ Urinalysis (*at diagnosis and yearly*)				
▪ Microalbuminuria (*Type1 puberty or after 5 years duration then yearly, Type 2 at dx then yearly)*				
▪ Creatinine Clearance and protein *(yearly after microalb > 300 mg/24hr)*				
▪ Ace Therapy *(if indicated*)				
CARDIOVASCULAR				
▪ Smoking status *(at each visit)*				
▪ Advised to quit smoking (*each visit)*				
▪ Smoking cessation referral *(if indicated*)				
▪ Lipid profile *(yearly)* TC/HDL/LDL/TG				
▪ Blood pressure (*each visit*)				
▪ Aspirin therapy *(if indicated*)				
▪ Review diet/weight goals (*each visit)*				
▪ Review physical activity (*each visit*)				
EYE CARE				
▪ Dilated eye exam (*Type 1 after 5 yrs duration, then yearly; Type 2 at diagnosis, then yearly)*				
FOOT CARE				
▪ Inspect bare feet and stress self exam (*each visit*)				
▪ Comprehensive lower extremity sensory exam *(yearly)*				
PREGNANCY				
▪ Assess contraception/discuss family planning *(at diagnosis and yearly during childbearing years)*				
NUTRITION THERAPY				
▪ At diagnosis, then Type 1: <18yoa every 3-6 mos, > 18yoa every 6-12 mos or as indicated. Type 2: every 6-12 mos or as indicated				
IMMUNIZATIONS				
▪ Influenza vaccine *(yearly)*				
▪ Pneumococcal vaccine *(once)*				

Form 20, Page 1

Educational Session/Physician Note Sample

Patient Name: Joe Smith **Date: 10/03/03**
Pharmacist: Smilie Smith, Pharm.D., CDE
Session Topic: Complications and Wrap-up

AREA EVALUATED	DENIES S/SX (X)	SIGNIFICANT FINDINGS
Chief Complaint		Patient just had an anal abscess drained today. He received treatment with Ciprofloxacin for 7 days, last tablet was 2 days ago. Denies any systemic sxs such as weakness or fever.
Hypoglycemia Dizziness - Trembling - Tachycardia - Sweating	X	
Hyperglycemia Polyphagia - Polydypsia - Polyuria - Nocturia	X	

REVIEW OF SYSTEMS	DENIES S/SX (X)	DOCUMENTATION
HEENT Dental caries - Infection - Bleeding - Ulcers - Visual changes	X	
CARDIOVASCULAR Chest discomfort - SOB - Pedal edema	X	
GU Urinary tract infection - Vaginal infection - Incontinence	X	
GI Diarrhea - Constipation - Gastroparesis - Flatulence		Anal abscess
NEUROLOGICAL Numbness - Tingling - Pain- Sexual dysfunction		He does have tingling in his feet which is less than when patient started the program.
FOOT CARE Callous - Cracking - Drying - Ulcers - Blisters	X	Wife does foot exam using the monofilaments on a daily basis.

MEDICAL CARE			
	Physician	Last Appointment	Next Appointment
Primary Care			
Endocrinologist			
Ophthalmologist			
Podiatrist			
Dentist			

DAILY ACTIVITY COMPLIANCE		
		Comments
Medication Regimen	X compliant noncompliant X changes ADR reported	Ciprofloxacin x 7 days
Dietary	Specific Diet X Yes No X ADA X Low-cholesterol X Low-salt Other Low in green vegetables containing Vitamin K Following dietary recommendations X Yes No	

Form 20, Page 2

Physical Activity	Type: None Frequency/Duration: ___ times/week for ___minutes Increased Decreased No change	
SMBG	X Yes No Frequency: TID to QID Timing: AM, lunch, dinner, and HS	
Foot Care	Wash daily X Yes No Inspect daily X Yes No	Wife is doing daily foot inspections.

SUBJECTIVE DATA

Patient denies any acute complaints except the pain at the site of the drainage. No bleeding or melena reported. No sxs of hypo or hyperglycemia. Patient has appointment at the A/C clinic at the VA hospital today.

OBJECTIVE DATA

Weight	X Increase Decrease No Change	259 lbs (increased by 3 lbs)
Blood Pressure	Increase Decrease X No Change	BP- 128/68
Pulse	78 R	
Finger Stick		

MEDICATIONS (including prescription, nonprescription, vitamins, and herbals)

Name	Dose	Indication	Prescriber	Start	Stop	Changes Y/N

ASSESSMENT/GOALS

Diabetes Control	Controlled Uncontrolled X Improved Worsened

Patient is asymptomatic and compliant to his medications. He is not taking any medications for diabetes and is controlling his diabetes with medical nutrition therapy. No side effects to the other medications he is receiving. Patient has already experienced some complications of diabetes such as neuropathy, retinopathy, and stroke. At the present time patient's medical conditions are controlled. Patient is willing to monitor on a regular basis and follow recommendations learned in the program to decrease the complications of diabetes and prevent further progression. We need to get the results of his last HbA1c to assess patient's overall glycemic long-term control.

An assessment of the patient's management skills for diabetes indicated that the patient achieved the outcome of the sessions. He has gained the knowledge and the skills to manage his diabetes effectively. Patient stated that the best thing about the program was the fact that by learning about his disease he was able to accept and cope with it.

Educational Session: Patient was educated about the acute and chronic complications of diabetes. Self-management skills for the prevention and control of complications caused by diabetes were discussed.

PLAN

1. Continue with current regimen.
2. Continue monitoring at least 2 x a day (AM fasting and another randomly before meals or at bedtime).
3. Patient will be f/u for the 3-month appointment in January 2004.
4. Long-term goals were developed (See wrap-up note)
5. Need lab data including renal function, cholesterol, urinalysis, BUN/Cr, and HbA1c.

Form 21, Page 1

Educational Session/Physician Note Blank

Patient Name: **Date:**
Pharmacist:
Session Topic:

AREA EVALUATED	DENIES S/SX (X)	SIGNIFICANT FINDINGS
Chief Complaint		
Hypoglycemia Dizziness - Trembling - Tachycardia - Sweating		
Hyperglycemia Polyphagia - Polydypsia - Polyuria - Nocturia		

REVIEW OF SYSTEMS	DENIES S/SX (X)	DOCUMENTATION
HEENT Dental caries - Infection - Bleeding - Ulcers - Visual changes		
CARDIOVASCULAR Chest discomfort - SOB - Pedal edema		
GU Urinary tract infection - Vaginal infection - Incontinence		
GI Diarrhea - Constipation - Gastroparesis - Flatulence		
NEUROLOGICAL Numbness - Tingling - Pain - Sexual dysfunction		
FOOT CARE Callous - Cracking - Drying - Ulcers - Blisters		

MEDICAL CARE			
Physician		Last Appointment	Next Appointment
Primary Care			
Endocrinologist			
Ophthalmologist			
Podiatrist			
Dentist			

DAILY ACTIVITY COMPLIANCE		
		Comments
Medication Regimen	compliant noncompliant changes ADR reported	
Dietary	Specific Diet Yes No ADA Low-cholesterol Low-salt Other ____________ Following dietary recommendations Yes No	

Form 21, Page 2

Physical Activity	Type: None Frequency/Duration: ___ times/week for ___minutes Increased Decreased No change	
SMBG	Yes No Frequency: TID to QID Timing: AM, lunch, dinner, and HS	
Foot Care	Wash daily Yes No Inspect daily Yes No	

SUBJECTIVE DATA

OBJECTIVE DATA		
Weight	Increase Decrease No Change	
Blood Pressure	Increase Decrease No Change	
Pulse		
Finger Stick		

MEDICATIONS (including prescription, nonprescription, vitamins, and herbals)

Name	**Dose**	**Indication**	**Prescriber**	**Start**	**Stop**	**Changes Y/N**

ASSESSMENT/GOALS	
Diabetes Control	Controlled Uncontrolled Improved Worsened
Educational Session:	

PLAN

Form 22

Quality Assurance Checklist

DATE________ REVIEWER'S INITIALS______ SATISFACTORY?	YES	NO
Initial assessment and checklist completed		
Chart contains physician referral for program		
Chart contains signed information disclosure consent form		
Chart contains completed medical history form		
Quality of life survey administered		
Knowledge questionnaire given		
Foot screening completed		
Appropriate lab work performed		
Monitoring flow sheet completed		
Patient goals established		
Assessment form faxed to primary care physician		
Chart contains physician letter from dietitian		
Final assessment and checklist completed		
Quality of life survey administered		
Knowledge questionnaire given		
Final lab work performed as appropriate		
Monitoring flow sheet completed		
Patient goals reviewed and assessed		
Assessment form faxed to primary care physician		

Notes:____

____

Appendix B

SAMPLE DOCUMENTS

Document 1

Program Description: Diabetes Care Program

The Diabetes Care Program at Caring Pharmacy offers comprehensive diabetes services to patients at two sites in the Paradise area. The program was developed as a partnership between the pharmacy and the University of Paradise School of Pharmacy. Instruction is offered to adults with Type 1 or Type 2 diabetes and their families.

The program offers individual one-on-one and group diabetes education, with participants attending eight 40- to 60-minute education sessions and two 30-minute follow-up sessions. The follow-up sessions are free of charge and are scheduled shortly (1 or 2 weeks) after completing the education sessions, and at 3 and 6 months later. The program is offered 2 days a week from 2 pm to 7 pm at each site, and the sessions are scheduled at the patient's convenience when possible.

Participants enter the program through self-referral, pharmacist referral, or physician referral. Potential participants are offered a free 15-minute initial consultation session to learn more about the program and discuss the benefits of participating. Once the patient is enrolled, his or her physician is notified of the program's goals and objectives and the qualifications of the staff educators. The physician is also asked to provide specific medical information as well as goals for the patient's diabetes care. During the initial educational session, the educator and participant use the information collected from the patient and the health care provider(s) to develop individualized educational and behavioral goals.

Specially trained pharmacists, nutritionists, and a certified diabetes educator provide the education sessions. A nutritionist meets with each participant and develops individualized meal plans. The pharmacists and the certified diabetes educator provide all other education sessions. Each participant receives a variety of written educational materials with each session, and those patients not monitoring blood glucose at home are given a meter free of charge.

Before and after each session, the educator assesses the participant's knowledge and skill level in the areas covered and documents achievement of the objectives. The patient and the educator select clinical and behavioral goals at the first session, based on patient preferences, needs, and lifestyle. These goals are reviewed and assessed at the beginning and the end of each session. If the goals are not being met, the educator discusses reasons for not meeting them and determines ways to overcome barriers. At each subsequent session the particular areas requiring improvement are addressed. After every session the patient's physician is informed about his or her progress in achieving the established goals, and is also made aware of any health-related issues identified and discussed in the session. Recommendations regarding the patient's diabetes care are also made to the physician as necessary after each session.

The program combines the expertise of the pharmacists on drug therapy issues and the convenience of a community pharmacy setting to offer a comprehensive service that provides many benefits beyond education. At the start of each session the patient's medication profile is reviewed and assessed for adherence, tolerability, and adverse effects. Objective data including blood pressure, pulse, and weight are obtained at each session as well. The pharmacist and the patient

continued on page 84

Document 1. Program Description: Diabetes Care Program, continued

review and discuss blood glucose readings obtained at home, and comorbidities that relate to diabetes care (i.e., hypertension, hyperlipidemia, obesity, coronary artery disease) are evaluated and addressed. In addition the participants discuss other individual health concerns, whether related to diabetes or not. All these findings are reported to the patient's physician in a written note so that problems can be addressed at the next visit.

A certified diabetes educator who is a faculty member at the University of Paradise School of Pharmacy coordinates the program. The coordinator meets on a weekly basis with the Manager of Pharmacy Services from Caring Pharmacy, Inc., to report program-related issues. All program staff report to the Program Coordinator.

The Program Coordinator and the Manager of Pharmacy Services at Caring pharmacy have selected the Advisory Committee members. The Advisory Committee is composed of faculty from the University of Paradise, Caring Pharmacy customers, program instructors, behavioral specialists, physicians, nurses, nutritionists, patients with diabetes who attended the program, and members of a major health insurance organization that provides medical coverage to a large percentage of Caring Pharmacy customers. The committee meets quarterly to discuss program issues and make recommendations to the Program Coordinator and sponsoring organization.

To assure quality of services, frequent meetings take place between the coordinator and the educators to assess issues related to the delivery of services, marketing of the program, and patient care. Recommendations of these meetings are implemented and reassessed at subsequent meetings.

Document 2

Program Description: Living Healthy with Diabetes

"Living Healthy with Diabetes" program at Caring Pharmacy offers comprehensive diabetes services to patients and their families in the Paradise Island and surrounding areas. This is one of the newest additions to the wellness services that Caring Pharmacy has traditionally offered to patients. Instruction—both group classes and one-on-one sessions—is offered to children and adults with Type 1 and Type 2 or gestational diabetes. Based on initial patient assessment and the needs of each patient, the educator enrolls the patient in a mix of classroom education and individual sessions. All pediatric and gestational patients receive mostly individual instruction.

Participants may enter the program through referral from their primary care provider, referral from other pharmacies, or self-referral. After initial assessment, the educator and patient discuss areas of need and collaborate to develop an individual education plan. A nurse educator, dietitians, pharmacists, physicians, and medical and pharmacy residents provide classroom and individual instruction.

All participants meet individually with a pharmacist to demonstrate diabetes knowledge and skills and also with a dietitian to develop an individualized meal plan. The main series of seven classes is offered at each site once every 3-4 months. Two sessions of each class run simultaneously at different times of the week to give patients flexibility in attending the sessions. Each site's series of classes is staggered by approximately 2 weeks to facilitate scheduling instructors. (The number of classes available at any given time may change according to need.)

On completion of the instruction, the educator will assess the participant's knowledge and skill level in each content area. If the participant is not competent, additional individual sessions may be needed until objectives are met. After the formalized program is completed, a tentative follow-up regimen is planned and further goals established for the patient. During follow-up, patients meet individually as needed with the educator, who reviews the patient's progress toward personal goals and reassesses overall diabetes control and drug therapy.

In addition to educating program participants, this program seeks to better manage the patient's overall diabetes control. During individual sessions with the educator, the patient's drug therapy will be assessed for appropriateness, necessary lab work will be obtained, and the primary care provider will be contacted if a problem arises. If needed, lab work will be obtained from the primary care provider or obtained directly at the pharmacy. The educator will collaborate with the primary care provider to meet the goals of the patient and physician and to comply with American Diabetes Association guidelines. Pertinent information will be sent back on a regular basis to inform the primary care provider of the patient's progress toward established goals. This program will not circumvent primary care providers but rather augment their efforts to achieve optimal outcomes for the patient.

The "Living Healthy with Diabetes" program has several unique qualities. The pharmacy location provides a convenient, accessible, and pleasing atmosphere for patient education. Many times, patients already have a relationship with some of the program instructors. Since the pharmacies are located in a grocery store setting, proper food choices can be easily demonstrated and grocery tours can be conducted.

Combining the education component with overall health management will lead to better patient outcomes than either option individually, and the multidisciplinary team approach will improve the process.

This program is sponsored by Caring Supermarkets, Inc. The coordinator reports to the Director of Pharmacy and Health Services, who reports to the Vice President of Operations. The Vice President of Operations reports directly to the Chief Executive Officer. All program staff report directly to the Program Coordinator, who receives guidance and input from the Advisory Committee and also from faculty at the Paradise University School of Pharmacy. In addition, the program receives support and assistance from physicians and staff at Lack of Time Family Physicians in Paradise. We hope that everyone who comes in contact with our program has a positive and fulfilling experience.

Document 3

Policies and Procedures Manual

[Editor's Note: Because this is a sample document only, the specific forms referred to here do not actually appear in Appendix A of this book.]

Mission Statement: The "Living Healthy with Diabetes" program provides patients with diabetes and their families the skills and knowledge to appropriately manage their disease, with the goal of improving their overall quality of life.

Advisory Committee

Purpose: The Advisory Committee helps plan the overall diabetes self-management education and management program, recommends and approves policy, and reviews program performance annually.

Membership: The Advisory Committee includes health professionals and others interested in the care and education of people with diabetes. The permanent members of the committee include:

Program coordinator
Behavioral specialist
Pharmacist instructor
Nurse educator
Dietitian
Health insurance representative
Site representative
Physician
Person with Type 2 diabetes
Caring Pharmacy administration
Paradise School of Pharmacy
Pharmacy resident
Patient with diabetes who attended program
Endocrinologist
ADA chapter representative

The membership of this committee is subject to change as needed by the program coordinator, with consideration given to the American Diabetes Association guidelines for recognized education programs. The coordinator serves as chair of this committee. Meetings are held quarterly in the community room at Caring Pharmacy. Members are encouraged to attend all meetings but must attend at least two meetings per year.

Responsibilities: The committee is responsible for planning and reviewing the program annually. The specific responsibilities are outlined below.

1. **Planning**
   a. Review and recommend changes in program objectives, target audience, participant access mechanisms, instructional methods, program resources
   b. Approve the annual program plan
   c. Review, recommend changes, and approve the curriculum and educational materials
   d. Review, recommend changes, and approve the organizational chart
2. **Recommending policy**
   a. Approve new program policies and recommend changes in policies
   b. Recommend policy to the administration
   c. Provide follow-up on recommended and approved policies
3. **Reviewing program performance annually**
   a. Whether program objectives were met
   b. Comparison between target and actual audience
   c. Ease by which participants enter or access the program

continued on page 87

d. Program follow-up mechanisms (determining the percentage of participants who completed the program through final assessment)
e. Adequacy of program resources, including space, personnel, and budget
f. The curriculum, educational materials, and community resource list for accuracy, currency, and appropriateness for the target audience
g. Marketing strategies to the target population and any potential referral sources
h. Program effectiveness by evaluating the summary of behavior change goals and HbA1c

4. Recommending program modifications based on the results of the annual review

Program Coordinator

The function of the program coordinator is to chair the Advisory Committee and oversee all aspects of the diabetes education program. The coordinator will organize all Advisory Committee meetings and ensure that requirements for ADA recognition are being met. The coordinator will perform site visits and review charts quarterly to see that the program's policy and procedures are executed properly and to ensure continuous quality improvement. The coordinator will solicit feedback from the program educators at each site for quality improvement as well as process-related improvements. The program coordinator will prepare the program plan and yearly program summary for the Advisory Committee to review and approve. The program coordinator reports directly to the director of pharmacy services.

Education Component

TIMELINE

1. Assessments: ***Initial assessment*** is conducted subsequent to the patient's referral and prior to any class education received by the patient. ***Final assessment*** is conducted ***approximately 3 months*** after initial assessment, provided the patient has obtained the planned education. The final assessment serves as the transition point between the education component and the management component of the program.
2. Consultation: Individual consultation is conducted as needed after the initial assessment through the final assessment. These consultations, by pharmacist or dietitian, can be held concurrently with the group classes and may continue up to the final assessment as needed for follow-up. Once the final assessment has been completed, any consultation after that is categorized as part of the management program.
3. Classes: Classes are held over a 2-month period three to four times each year. During a single cycle, each class is given once or twice at each location with an effort to provide flexibility for patient scheduling.

STAFF

Various health care professionals—including but not limited to physicians, dietitians, pharmacists, and nurses—teach the group classes. Occasionally other types of instructors may teach portions of a class based on their expertise, such as fitness experts, psychologists, etc. Pharmacists and dietitians conduct most individual consultations. At least one pharmacist at each site has special diabetes training, and there are three dietitians available for consultations. All personnel labeled as program staff must complete certification or a certificate program along with continuing education in diabetes, as designated by the program coordinator.

PATIENT ENROLLMENT

- Patients are enrolled in a variety of ways.

  Patients may ***show interest in the program directly to the pharmacist*** or pharmacy or may ***be targeted by the pharmacist for participation***. This could happen at any of our pharmacy stores. Each store should fill out an Interest Form for interested patients and fax this form to the appropriate store that participates in the

continued on page 88

Document 3. Policies and Procedures Manual, continued

education program. Once payment arrangements are made, these patients are enrolled immediately. If needed, a referral from the patient's physician is obtained at this time.

- Patients may be ***referred to the pharmacy by their physician***. Once a referral is received, the pharmacist contacts the patient and starts the process. Once payment arrangements are made, these patients are enrolled. The Interest Form still needs to be filled out for these patients and kept in the chart.
- Patients may be ***referred to the pharmacy by their insurance company***. After the referral is received, if the patient does not initiate the first contact by 2 weeks before the classes start, the pharmacist calls the patient to enroll him or her in the program. Once the patient has made contact, the patient is handled as if he or she had been targeted by the pharmacist for participation.

Before the initial assessment it is necessary for the patient to fill out a Diabetes Medical History Form, Liability Waiver/Information Disclosure Consent Form and a Quality of Life Questionnaire. These must be returned to the pharmacist *before* the initial assessment visit to allow the pharmacist to review them before this appointment. Once the patient is enrolled, the pharmacist should fax the Interest Form and the specific classes each patient will be attending to the program coordinator for compilation.

COMPUTER PROGRAM

A tracking system is used to track patient education received and outcomes assessed for American Diabetes Association recognition. All patients enrolled in the education program are entered into the tracking system. **The patient's record in the tracking system is kept current by the educator at each individual visit.**

At the initial visit the following must be documented:

1. Demographic information
2. Assessment information
3. Education needed
4. Behavioral goals established
5. Initial physical assessment and laboratory information
6. Initial scoring on Knowledge Questionnaire and Quality of Life Questionnaire

At each routine visit the following must be documented:

1. Education the patient has received since the last visit
2. Assessment of progress toward goals
3. Physical assessment values, including laboratory values

At the final assessment the following must be documented:

1. Education the patient has received since the last visit
2. Assessment of progress toward goals
3. Physical assessment values, including laboratory values
4. Scoring of the final Knowledge Questionnaire and Quality of Life Questionnaire

At the time of applying or reapplying for ADA recognition, the program coordinator queries the computer program for necessary information and reports to submit to ADA.

PAYMENT

- Patients paying out of pocket for the program are charged the established fee and may opt to pay in two installments at the discretion of the pharmacist.

continued on page 89

Document 3. Policies and Procedures Manual, continued

- Third-party payers are billed in two ways:

1. According to any agreement that has been made.
2. The entire fee upon enrollment in the program. If the claim is rejected for a particular patient, that patient is billed for the service. Every attempt is made to obtain payment from a patient's third-party payer.

- Caring Pharmacy associates and their immediate family members receive the program at no cost as a covered benefit through Caring Pharmacy.

PHYSICIAN FOLLOW-UP

The patient's physician or other primary care provider is contacted several times throughout the course of the program.

- Initially, a letter is sent explaining the program and requesting a referral if one has not already been received from the physician.
- Once the patient completes the initial assessment, the physician receives a letter with the Initial Assessment Form, Patient Contract, and Information Disclosure Consent Form attached. This letter may include a request for laboratory information or even recommendations to maintain compliance with ADA guidelines, if appropriate.
- During the course of the classwork, after patients have visits with the pharmacist, the physician receives additional information.
- The dietitian sends the physician a summary of his or her visit with the patient.
- After the final assessment, the physician receives a letter detailing the classes that were attended. This letter may outline opportunities for the patient to improve diabetes control.

Communication occurs over 2 to 4 months and is meant to keep the physician informed of the patient's participation and progress through the program. These communications are tailored to meet the needs of particular physicians.

LAB WORK

Lab work is performed only when part of an investigational study, when not easily obtainable from the primary care provider's office, or when specifically requested by a payer. It is not the intent of this program to duplicate lab work. The Patient Monitoring Flowsheet is used to record lab work and other monitoring information, whether obtained at the pharmacy or elsewhere.

INITIAL ASSESSMENT

The initial assessment is the first appointment with the patient. The following goals are accomplished in 1 hour if possible. *To necessitate this, it is imperative that the pharmacist educator has reviewed the Medical History Form before the patient's appointment and that the patient has completed the necessary paperwork before the appointment.*

- The patient finishes any paperwork that has not been completed.
- The patient completes a Knowledge Questionnaire at this visit. This same questionnaire is given to the patient again at the final assessment.
- The pharmacist assesses the patient's knowledge in the 10 content areas established by the American Diabetes Association by talking with the patient as well as reviewing the Knowledge Questionnaire. This is documented on the back of the Initial Assessment Form.
- The pharmacist and patient decide which classes the patient will attend and how often to meet with the patient individually.
- The patient establishes behavioral goals with input from the pharmacist educator as well as from the physician.
- The pharmacist performs necessary lab work, depending on the patient's classification.

continued on page 90

Document 3. Policies and Procedures Manual, continued

Classes

As noted previously, patients are scheduled for classes based on their initial assessment. Classes are offered either once or twice per week depending on the demand at a particular site. Class times vary, depending on the location, to accommodate the vast majority of patients' needs. The first class in the series is generally taught by a physician in the community. The second and third classes are taught by the dietitian educator. The fourth through sixth classes are taught mainly by pharmacist educators, pharmacy residents, nurses, and Paradise School of Pharmacy faculty members. Occasionally, other specialists from the surrounding community teach all or part of some classes.

Following are responsibilities of the instructor for each individual class, with the exception of class #1. The primary pharmacist at each site is responsible for handling these duties for class #1.

- **All Classes:**
  - —The primary pharmacist will verify the availability of the community room before the class.
  - —Participants must sign the sign-in sheet to document attendance. There may be separate sign-in sheets for separate patient groups.
  - —The instructor must print and sign his or her name on this sign-in sheet as well.
  - —Each participant and guest must complete an evaluation form. The instructor will make a point of requesting suggestions for improving those items that were not scored at the highest rating.
  - —The primary pharmacist or dietitian will forward all evaluation forms to the program coordinator after each class.
  - —The primary pharmacist or dietitian will fax the sign-in sheet to the program coordinator immediately after each class.

- **Class #1:** Each participant is given a reference book, which is another source of information for the patient and is referenced throughout the series of classes.
- **Class #2**: Each participant is given a "Diabetes Shopping Guide."
- **Class #3:** At the conclusion of the third class each participant is asked to make an appointment with the dietitian by calling the nutrition hotline and is given a Food Journal Form to fill out before that appointment. That appointment, which is approximately 1 hour, is used to develop an individualized meal plan and suggest ways for the patient to improve his or her eating habits as they relate to diabetes.
- **Class #4:** During the fourth class, patients are given an application for membership in the American Diabetes Association and are supplied a copy of *Diabetes Forecast* to show them one of the many benefits of joining the ADA.
- **Class #5:** After this class the primary pharmacist will forward the names of participants to the program coordinator so that certificates of completion can be created.
- **Class #6:** The final class is used partly as a graduation. Each participant is given a certificate of completion and is included in a class photograph. This class may also be used for "show and tell" about meters and devices if the instructor wishes.

One of the goals of having patients participate in group classes is the bond formed among the participants and guests. Over this 6-week period, generally, patients see the same people at each class. Patients are encouraged to participate, ask questions, and share experiences at these classes, which helps patients get to know each other. This becomes a very positive experience for the participants and guests, and they are apt to learn more this way.

NUTRITION CONSULTATION

Included in the education component of the program is one hour-long session with the dietitian to answer specific questions and develop an individualized meal plan. During class #3 of the program, the dietitian informs participants of the availability of this session. Participants are asked to call the nutrition hotline to schedule this appointment.

continued on page 91

Document 3. Policies and Procedures Manual, continued

For stores without a staff dietitian, scheduling may be challenging. The dietitian responsible for these particular stores may set aside blocks of time, and at class #3 let patients know about these blocks so as to make the best use of the dietitian's time. The dietitian should make every attempt to meet with patients at their "home" store for these sessions.

The dietitian must review the nutrition information from the medical history form in the patient's chart before the appointment. After the appointment, a letter is sent to the patient's physician and a copy placed in the patient's diabetes chart. The dietitian notes the date of this session in the patient's chart on the Final Assessment Form . For statistical purposes, the dietitian makes note of the visit with the nutrition hotline. *It is ultimately the responsibility of the pharmacist educator to make sure patients are scheduling their dietitian appointments.* He or she can check in with patients about these appointments at the remaining group classes.

PHARMACIST CONSULTATION

Pharmacist educators schedule their patient appointments when it is convenient for both the pharmacist and the patient. It may be before or after a pharmacist's shift or during an overlap time period. Each time the pharmacist educator sees a patient, a Routine Assessment Form is filled out and inserted in the chart, and information is recorded in the tracking system, as noted previously. Patients are encouraged to bring their blood glucose monitors to these appointments to download into the computer. Reports of their blood glucose readings are kept in the chart and forwarded to the physician. Routine monitoring performed at each visit includes blood pressure, pulse, weight, and possibly blood glucose. Hemoglobin A1c measures and lipid profiles are performed only at the initial and follow-up assessments, and then only if needed. Each visit with the pharmacist educator is recorded on the Final Assessment Form, along with the number of hours spent at that appointment.

FINAL ASSESSMENT

Once the patient has completed the assigned classes and the recommended dietitian and pharmacist individual visits, the pharmacist schedules a final assessment session. Much like the initial assessment, this session focuses on evaluating the patient's knowledge.

- The pharmacist educator uses the Final Assessment Form to guide him or her through the final assessment.
- The patient is asked to complete the Knowledge Questionnaire and the Quality of Life Questionnaire, just as he or she did in the initial assessment.
- Lab work is performed if necessary.
- Goals that were set in the beginning are reviewed. Based on the percent completion of these goals, the pharmacist and patient work together to set new goals to help the patient to continue managing his or her diabetes.

The final assessment marks the end of the education component of the program and the beginning of the management and follow-up component. Recording the date of this transition in the tracking system is crucial.

QUALITY IMPROVEMENT

To monitor continuous quality improvement, the following steps must be taken:

- The program coordinator continually evaluates patient progress with input from the staff educators and administration.
- The advisory committee, which meets quarterly, also has input as follows.
  —Behavioral outcome measures, which are recorded in the tracking software, are monitored on a quarterly basis coinciding with each advisory committee meeting. The behavioral outcomes measured depend on the patient, but may include nutritional management; physical activity; medications; monitoring, preventing, detecting, and treating complications; risk reduction; or psychosocial adjustment.

continued on page 92

Document 3. Policies and Procedures Manual, continued

—Health outcome measures recorded in the tracking software are monitored quarterly, coinciding with each Advisory Committee meeting. The health outcomes measured in all patients are HbA1c, eye exams, quality of life, and foot exams.

—Results from an annual patient satisfaction survey, which is mailed to past participants, are reviewed.

- Patient charts are reviewed on an ongoing basis by both the program coordinator and by Paradise School of Pharmacy faculty. Ten percent of the charts at each site are reviewed quarterly.
- All class evaluation forms from each site are compiled and evaluated after each session for quality improvement of the classes. These results are reported to the Advisory Committee.

The Advisory Committee considers all this information and, at its annual program review, recommends changes for correcting deficiencies in any of the mentioned areas, as well as the means by which these changes will be implemented.

Management Component

Once enrolled in the management component of the program, patients will be seen or contacted at least once every 3 months to obtain information, assess continued progress toward goals, answer questions, and communicate information to the physician. These sessions should last approximately 20 to 30 minutes each. The execution of this management component will be based on compensation for these services by the patient or third party. It is the goal of this program to continue to follow those patients who have been educated to assess their continued success in managing their disease and to determine when additional education may be necessary. Ongoing follow-up will ultimately keep the diabetes patient healthy and limit the disease complications.

STAFF

Staff for the management component of the program is essentially the same as for the education component.

SCHEDULING

Patients are scheduled for management visits subsequent to their follow-up assessment.

PAPERWORK

At each management visit, the pharmacist educator uses the Routine Assessment Form to document that visit, and keeps a copy in the chart.

LABORATORY TESTS

Laboratory test are performed only if not being done by the patient's physician.

PHYSICIAN FOLLOW-UP

The patient's physician will be notified if there are any problems that are identified as a result of these management visits.

Document 4

Annual Program Plan: May 2002-April 2003

Diabetes Care Program

Statement of Support

The Board of Directors of Caring Pharmacy, Inc., strongly believes that self-management education is an integral component of the appropriate care of people with diabetes. We continue to support the staff and their commitment to improve the lives of people with diabetes. The Diabetes Care Program is an integral part of our new Wellness Initiative aimed at improving the lives and health of our clients.

Based on the annual program review, the Caring Pharmacy Diabetes Care Program will continue to offer a uniquely comprehensive diabetes education program to adult customers with Type 1 and Type 2 diabetes and their families.

Instructional Methods

Includes individual sessions with demonstrations and graphic presentations. Participant involvement and self-motivation are encouraged through individual needs assessment and goal setting. The participant, with guidance and support from the educator and physicians, helps determine the order of educational modules and frequency of visits. The use of videotapes and group sessions will be implemented later this year.

Target Population

All adult patients ($\geq$ 18 years old) with diabetes (Type 1 and Type 2) and their families. Patients with gestational diabetes are not included in the program. Our service area includes the Heart and Love area in Pleasantville. There are approximately 800 patients with diabetes in the service area, based on prescription drug records. The language is predominantly English with a small percent of Spanish, Korean, and Vietnamese-speaking participants in the Love area. Sites are located in multiethnic suburban to urban communities with African-American and Hispanic groups. The population is diverse in ethnic makeup, educational level, and socioeconomic status.

PARTICIPANTS' ACCESS MECHANISMS

Participants access the program through physicians, pharmacists, or self-referral. During the first year of the program's existence there have been no problems with participant access.

FOLLOW-UP

Participants will be followed up at 3 and 6 months after completing the entire program. If a participant is unable to keep the follow-up appointment, a telephone assessment will be done within 2 weeks by a staff member of the diabetes care program. The follow-up visit or telephone contact will include an assessment of health status, knowledge, skills and attitudes, behavioral goals, and post-program adherence with diabetes medications, daily foot examination, and self-blood glucose measurements. Follow-up rates have been good based on results of the annual program review, and no changes in the follow-up mechanisms are needed. A new documentation form will be used to document attainment of goals.

continued on page 94

Document 4. Annual Program Plan: May 2002-April 2003, Diabetes Care Program, continued

Resource Requirements

The private counseling rooms currently used are adequate for individual sessions. A waiting room is available. The current staff of at least two pharmacists and one dietitian as program instructors at each site has met the needs of enrolled patients. We will explore facilities for group sessions, to meet the needs of the Medicare population. A VCR and TV are needed to use videocassettes in the educational sessions.

Outcome Measure(s) Chosen and Means of Evaluating

Besides tracking participant's achievement of educational goals, the program has tracked glycemic control based on hemoglobin A1c, percentage of patients having annual dilated retinal eye exams, percentage of patients performing daily foot exam, and self-blood glucose measurement pre- and post-program. The results of these outcome measures were reported to the Advisory Committee during the annual review in January 2002. Based on the findings of the annual review and the discussion of the committee, the program objectives will be the same, although the wording of various objectives will be modified slightly. The new objectives for the year 2002 are as follows:

CLINICAL

1. To reduce individual HbA1c once diagnosed with diabetes by 1% in a 12-month period, unless the patient is already within the target range.
2. To increase by 20% the number of participants who have an annual dilated retinal exam by increasing visits to the ophthalmologist.

BEHAVIORAL

1. To increase by 20% the percentage of program participants performing a daily foot exam.
2. To increase by 20% the percentage of participants who monitor blood glucose at home regularly. Also, to provide a meter to all participants who don't already have one free of charge.

ADMINISTRATIVE

1. Increase the number of program participants to 30 a year per site by increasing marketing of the program through scheduling visits to physician offices and advertising in local newspapers.
2. Develop a condensed program to reduce the number of educational sessions from eight to four to reduce participants' time commitment.
3. Obtain educational materials written in Korean and Vietnamese.
4. Explore the feasibility of using videotaped and group components in addition to individual live education sessions.

The annual program plan for 2002-2003 is approved by the Advisory Committee and Caring Pharmacy, Inc., March 23, 2002.

_______________	_______________
Date	Program Coordinator Chair, Advisory Committee
_______________	_______________
Date	Vice President, Pharmacy Operations Caring Pharmacy, Inc.

Document 5

Giant Diabetes Education Program Curriculum

OUTLINE FOR THE PHARMACIST

1. Introduction

a. Ask patient if they have questions or concerns from last session. Answer questions and address any concerns.
b. Summarize briefly the important concepts from last session and review short-term goals.
c. Ask if patient discussed last session with physician. Record any patient comments.
d. Collect any new information from patient.

2. Data Collection Process

a. Pharmaceutical Care Database—collect information regarding complications, signs and symptoms of complications, recent episodes of hypo/hyperglycemia, recent illnesses.
b. Review patient's medications. If there are changes from the last session, assess for drug interactions, ADRs, and compliance.
c. Collect and record necessary related objective data: blood pressure, weight, foot exam, signs and symptoms of complications, glucose readings, etc.

3. Module II – Monitoring

a. Follow instructions in session binder – NOTE: Provide appropriate information from curriculum according to patient's individual needs and type of diabetes. Eliminate unnecessary information and highlight particularly pertinent information.
b. Provide take-home educational materials.
c. Allow patient to ask questions.

4. Goal Setting

a. Review short-term and long-term goals with the patient.

5. Fill out follow-up form for patient with the return date and record in the appointment book.

6. Write the physician note within 24 hours of patient visit.

7. Fax and/or mail summary note to the physician.

8. File patient's chart in filing cabinet alphabetically.

Source: Developed by Magaly Rodriguez de Bittner and used with permission from Giant Pharmacy.

Document 6

Giant Diabetes Education Program Module II: Monitoring

Statement of Purpose

This session is intended to provide information about monitoring issues, management options, and therapy relationships that are important for a patient with diabetes to understand. Patients will learn how to monitor using a glucometer and how to understand the relationship of the glucose level with nutrition, drug therapy, stress, and exercise. They will learn appropriate self-management techniques.

Educational Objectives

At the completion of this module, the patient should be able to:

1. Explain that blood is tested to determine the actual level of glucose in the blood.
2. List different methods of testing blood glucose and state the value of blood glucose testing over urine testing.
3. Demonstrate recommended self-monitoring blood glucose (SMBG) technique and demonstrate how to interpret the results.
4. Explain the importance of maintaining a complete diabetes record (SMBG logbook).
5. List personal benefits of monitoring blood glucose levels.
6. Identify when and how to perform maintenance/repairs to their blood glucose meters.
7. List necessary supplies to conduct SMBG.
8. List at least four factors that can affect the results of blood tests.
9. State the purpose, importance, and implications of HbA1c monitoring and value.
10. State when to test blood glucose and urine ketones.
11. List resources available to help patients with their monitoring efforts and glucose meter use.
12. Describe the relationship between nutrition, exercise, medications, and monitoring of blood glucose and HbA1c, and their effects on blood glucose.
13. Identify patterns and trends in their blood glucose levels, especially as they relate to therapy.
14. Make an assessment of why these trends or patterns may be developing, and develop appropriate action to take.
15. Understand how adequate blood glucose control influences the development and progression of acute and chronic complications, and relate this effect to the findings of the Diabetes Control and Complications Trial (DCCT) and the United Kingdom Prospective Diabetes Study (UKPDS) trials.
16. Identify members of the interdisciplinary team and their respective roles in the patient's overall management and monitoring plan.

CONTENT OUTLINE

The pharmacist should discuss the following points:

I. Self-monitoring Blood Glucose/HbA1c

1. Need and benefits of SMBG.
2. Overview of different glucose meters and selection of the one that meets the patient's needs.
3. Overview of proper use/maintenance of meter.
4. Development of a personal monitoring plan for the patient including testing technique, frequency of testing, development of a SMBG logbook, and interpretation of the results.
5. Availability of additional products necessary to adequately self-monitor purpose, importance, frequency, implications, and use of the HbA1c value.

continued on page 97

Document 6. Giant Diabetes Education Program Module II: Monitoring, continued

6. Discussion of situations when urine glucose/ketone/protein testing may be warranted and how to interpret the results.
7. Discussion of resources available to assist the patient in self-monitoring efforts (e.g., toll-free numbers, manufacturer resources, pamphlets, support groups).

II. Therapy Relationships

1. Review the relationships among nutrition, exercise, medication, and self-monitoring and the effects of each of these on blood glucose levels.
2. Review the patient's self-monitoring diary and teach the patient how to recognize trends and patterns in blood glucose and their association with nonpharmacological and pharmacological therapy (if applicable).
3. Instruct how to identify possible reasons for trends in blood glucose values.
4. Review recommended and personal target glucose/HbA1c ranges and identify critical levels when the patient should contact his or her health care provider or seek immediate care.
5. Reinforce need to self-monitor for symptoms and blood glucose level to identify problem areas in their care.

III. Management Options

1. The effects of adequate blood glucose control on acute and long-term complications of diabetes.
2. The basic design of the DCCT and the UKPDS, and their findings.
3. The members of the health care team and their respective roles.
4. Recommended target blood glucose levels and HbA1c values.

EDUCATIONAL METHODS AND MATERIALS

Methods:

Discussion, demonstration

Materials:

—Boehringer Mannheim, *Use of Results, Hemoglobin A1c, Ketone Testing (for Type 1 patients), Blood Glucose Monitoring*
—Novo-Nordisk, *Understanding glycosylated hemoglobin*
—PACE Diabetes Program, *What is your number?*
—Self-monitoring logbook

Evaluation Plan

Knowledge will be evaluated by achievement of learning objectives and by responses to questions during the session. The ability to apply knowledge will be evaluated by the development of self-management goals, by the development and implementation of a plan, and through the program outcome measures.

The learning outcomes will be evaluated at the beginning of the following session to assess whether patients achieved the outcomes. If not, a review will take place with further evaluation at a later day.

Documentation Plan

Outcomes will be recorded in the outcome assessment form for each patient.

Clinical data and pharmacist's recommendations will go on the designated patient information forms. Documentation forms will be kept in the patient file and maintained in the file cabinet.

Source: Developed by Magaly Rodriguez de Bittner and used with permission from Giant Pharmacy.

Document 7

Giant Diabetes Education Program Content Outline

Concept	Information	Instructor's Notes
1. Purpose of testing	**1.1** Monitoring your blood and urine for ketones (in the case of a Type 1 patient) gives you valuable information about your blood glucose level and the effects of meal patterns, food intake, medication, activity, and stress.	Ask the patient ***Are you monitoring your blood glucose?*** ***How are you monitoring it?*** ***How frequently?***
	1.2 Level of glucose in the blood results from interaction of: meals, medications for diabetes, physical activity, and stress. They change throughout the day and night.	Give examples of how monitoring data can be recorded in daily self-care.
2. Methods used to monitor diabetes control	**2.1** Keeping a diabetes record helps you track your glucose level. This helps you use this information more easily and helps your physician treat your diabetes more effectively.	
	2.2 Testing your blood is a direct method that tells you exactly how much glucose is in your bloodstream. It is the recommended method to monitor your glucose.	
	2.3 Urine testing is an indirect method to test for blood glucose and ketones (if you use the ketone test). It is not as accurate and it is not recommended unless blood testing cannot be performed. Ketones are still tested in the urine if the blood glucose level is elevated (usually when it exceeds 240 mg/dL or during sick days). This is recommended in Type 1 patients because they are prone to diabetes ketoacidosis.	Ask the patient ***Do you know your HbA1c or glycosylated hemoglobin level?*** ***Have you ever had this test done?***
	2.4 An additional test, usually done in the hospital laboratory or some physician's offices, is the HbA1c or glycosylated hemoglobin test. This test tells us the amount of glucose attached to the hemoglobin in the red blood cell. (This is different from the test done for iron deficiency or anemia.)	Show picture of glycosylated hemoglobin. Give patient Novo-Nordisk pamphlet on HbA1c.

continued on page 99

Document 7. Giant Diabetes Education Program Content Outline, continued

Concept	Information	Instructor's Notes
	2.5 This test indicates the level of control over the previous 3-4 months. It measures the average blood glucose level over a period of time. It tells control over time. It can be done with a laboratory test or a fingerstick.	Each laboratory has its normal ranges. Recommend that the patient inquire about this test and try to get it done every 3-6 months depending on his/her level of glucose control or the availability of the test.
	2.6 It gives the big picture of your blood glucose control, while a blood glucose test gives you a snapshot at that moment. Your red blood cells carry the memory of all your blood glucose levels over the 3-month period.	
	2.7 Your glycosylated hemoglobin reading is not a simple average, but a weighted average. You never have a complete turnover of all red blood cells. About half were formed during the last month. So your glucose levels in the last month count for about half of your glycosylated hemoglobin (HbA1c) measurement, and red blood cells from the previous 2-3 months make up the other half of the measurement.	Ask ***Did your doctor discuss with you your goals for glycosylated hemoglobin?*** Show diagram, "Regulating Blood Glucose."
	2.8 Research has demonstrated that long-term control is important. Keeping HbA1c levels at 7% or lower helps prevent or delay the long-term complications of diabetes. **In some circumstances, physicians may determine in consultation with the patient a different goal, based on the patient's medical conditions or his or her inability to meet this goal**.	
	2.9 There is an additional test, fructosamine, that measures blood glucose control over the previous 2-3 weeks. It indicates short-term control. It is used less frequently but is an alternative when HbA1c cannot be done. Some glucometers monitor both blood glucose and fructosamine.	

continued on page 100

Document 7. Giant Diabetes Education Program Content Outline, continued

Concept	Information	Instructor's Notes
3.Choosing a glucose testing method	**3.1** Levels of glucose in the blood result from interaction of: meal plan, medicines for diabetes, exercise, and stress	Ask ***What would you expect your glucose to do 1 hour after you eat?***
	3.2 Glucose levels change throughout the day and night	Ask ***What is normal blood glucose?*** Note that blood glucose levels nearer the normal range help to prevent complications.
	3.3 You need to set personal blood glucose goals with your health care team. These goals may change from time to time. You'li use these goals as a guide for using your monitoring data.	Ask the patient to show you the meter he or she is currently using. If the patient does not have one, ask appropriate questions to help select a meter for the patient.
	3.4 There are two major methods of blood glucose testing: meter-read test strips and visually read test strips. Preferred method is the meter-read. There is less opportunity for misinterpretation by the patient.	Show the patient examples of various meters and explain the differences among them.
	3.5 These tests require a drop of blood. Noninvasive meters have been developed but they are not available yet. It is unknown when they will be on the market.	Ask ***Has your physician recommended a specific meter?***
	3.6 There are many different meters available. They vary in features, portability, and cost.	Specific technique for the meter chosen will be discussed during the testing session. At this time, put other meters away and keep the one the patient has selected based on his or her needs.
	3.7 Choice of the meter is based on the specific characteristics of the patient, on personal preference, cost, features (e.g., memory), ease of use, and in some cases, what is covered by insurance companies. Sometimes health insurance companies have special contracts that require using a particular type of meter.	Show examples of computer printouts if available. Ask patients if they have a computer. What about their physician—do they have a program to download this information?
	3.8 Some meters have computer programs that allow patients and their health care providers to download the results from their meters' memory to a computer. This allows the results to be printed and plotted in a graph format.	Show examples of test strips and stress the importance of waiting the recommended amount of time before comparing the results to the chart. Visual strips can be more expensive that the strips for the meters.

continued on page 101

Document 7. Giant Diabetes Education Program Content Outline, continued

Concept	Information	Instructor's Notes
	3.9 Visual-read strips have an enzyme that reacts with glucose levels and changes color. After a specific period of time, the color of the strip is compared to a color chart to determine the level of glucose.	
4. When to test and how frequently	**4.1** When to test is based on the treatment, level of blood glucose, goals, and symptoms. **4.2** There are many options for testing. Testing blood glucose at various times of the day gives a better picture of control than testing only once a day after fasting. You may use one or more of these options: ■ 1-8 times a day ■ before each meal and at bedtime ■ fasting and 2 hours after each meal ■ before and after each meal ■ once a day, but at different times each day (e.g., Monday before breakfast, Tuesday at bedtime, etc.) ■ fasting and once more at a different time of the day (as above) ■ each day before breakfast ■ fasting, before dinner, and at bedtime. **4.3** Test more frequently (every 2-4 hours) when ill, especially patients using insulin or Type 1 patients.	Ask ***How often do you test?*** Ask ***How often do you think you need to test to achieve your blood glucose goals?*** Postprandial testing is recommended in people using Lispro or a carbohydrate uptake inhibitor, acarbose, or when there is a discrepancy between fasting glucose and HbA1c.
5. Recording and interpreting	**5.1** Write down the results of your tests in a logbook. These logbooks are provided to patients free of charge. Bring the results to your appointments along with the monitor. **5.2** If your glucometer has extended memory you do not have to write the test unless you want to. It is beneficial if you lose the meter or the glucometer malfunctions (battery or other issues).	

continued on page 102

Document 7. Giant Diabetes Education Program Content Outline, continued

Concept	Information	Instructor's Notes
	5.3 You need to decide personal benefits of monitoring.	
	5.4 Monitoring alone will not control your glucose. You can use the results of your tests to adjust your meal plan, medicine, and exercise.	
	5.5 Look for patterns in your blood glucose levels. Think about possible causes for your blood glucose patterns or changes from your usual patterns. This is the first step in using the results.	
	5.6 Call your doctor or health care provider if any problems arise between visits or if there are major changes in your results. Also call if you have low blood glucose reactions for reasons you do not understand, or if your blood glucose levels change suddenly and you do not know why or what to do.	
	5.7 It is important to keep careful and accurate records. Always write the time of the test and the relationship with meals and medications. You may want to also record any dietary changes that may explain the results of a particular test.	
	5.8 It is important to have your individual blood glucose levels and know when to contact your physician or health care provider.	
	5.9 ADA-recommended goals: ■ Fasting: 80-120 mg/dL ■ Postprandial: < 180 mg/dL ■ Bedtime: 100-140 mg/dL These goals may be different in a particular patient. It is important to set these goals with your physician.	

continued on page 103

Document 7. Giant Diabetes Education Program Content Outline, continued

Concept	Information	Instructor's Notes
	5.10 The DCCT trial demonstrated that if blood glucose levels are maintained between these recommended ranges the long-term complications of diabetes can be delayed or prevented.	
6. How to do blood glucose testing	**6.1** Blood glucose testing may seem hard to do at first. As you learn to use the results to understand your body better and control your blood glucose, it will become easier. **6.2** Before you do the test, gather all your materials and get them in order. You may want to get your testing equipment in a small box (could use a shoebox) or bag so that the materials are stored together. **6.3** Keep the testing material near the place you usually test so it will take less time. Keep your diabetes record and a pen in the same place. **6.4** Plan ways to make testing part of your daily routine. **6.5** To obtain an adequate drop of blood: ■ Wash your hands in warm water before finger prick. ■ Dangle the fingers at your side before finger prick. ■ Squeeze below the place on your finger where you are going to prick until it turns red. ■ Prick the sides of your fingertips, not the fatty middle part. ■ Keep your hands below the level of your heart while you wait for the drop to reach an adequate size. ■ Gently milk your fingers. ■ Try your thumb or fourth finger—they have a rich blood supply.	Ask ***What do you learn by testing?***

continued on page 104

Document 7. Giant Diabetes Education Program Content Outline, continued

Concept	Information	Instructor's Notes
	6.6 Do not use monitoring equipment that belongs to another person, and avoid sharing your equipment with others. This prevents the transmission of infections and diseases. **6.7** Evaluate the results and use them to adjust your insulin, meal plan, or activity level if instructed by your physician. **6.8** Reward yourself for testing and recording your blood results.	
7. Factors that affect blood glucose test results	**7.1** Factors that affect your blood glucose level: ■ Food and beverages ■ Medicine for diabetes ■ Other medicines ■ Exercise ■ Stress ■ Timing of food and diabetes medication ■ Time of day the test is performed **7.2** Outdated strips: check expiration date. **7.3** Technique errors: ■ Collection methods ■ Inadequate blood sample ■ Meter not correctly calibrated to strips ■ Meter needs to be cleaned ■ Need new batteries **7.4** Meter malfunction.	Ask the patient ***What factors can affect blood glucose level?*** ***If these factors happened to you can you share with us how you dealt with them?*** Store materials in a cool, dry place. Heat and dampness can affect the test materials. Check the directions for the meter. If it still does not work, contact the manufacturer's toll free number.
8. Ketone testing	**8.1** Ketones appear in the urine when the body cells do not have enough glucose to use for energy because there is: ■ Not enough insulin activity due to inadequate dose of the medication or illness ■ Not enough food, as in a weight-loss diet or with hypoglycemia.	**Present this section only if Type 1 patients.** Ask the patient ***What are ketones?*** Blood glucose tests do not provide information about ketones. Urine tests are needed for ketone results.

continued on page 105

Document 7. Giant Diabetes Education Program Content Outline, continued

Concept	Information	Instructor's Notes
	8.2 The body burns fat for energy when glucose is not available. Ketones are a waste product of this fat metabolism.	Show examples of various strips.
	8.3 Ketones are acid. Buildup of ketones upsets the body's balance and ketoacidosis results.	Present information specific to the patient.
	8.4 Several products are on the market to test for ketones.	
	8.5 Urine tests reflect the amount of ketones in the blood during the time the urine was made by the kidneys.	Ketoacidosis is rare in Type 2 patients.
	8.6 When to test for ketones: ■ IF Type 1: whenever your blood glucose is over 240 mg/dL; whenever you feel ill; early-morning tests can tell you if you had a reaction during the night ■ IF Type 2 (especially if using insulin): whenever you feel sick or when the blood glucose is running high (around 300) most of the time.	These are early signs of diabetic ketoacidosis.
	8.7 Interpretation of results of ketone tests: ■ If ketone results are positive, drink water or other sugar-free drinks. ■ Call your health care provider to let him or her know and get instructions on what to do next. ■ Test blood glucose and urine ketones every 2 hours until normal.	Monitoring can provide flexibility by increasing the ability to make adjustments and decisions. A blood glucose level below 70 mg/dL generally indicates hypoglycemia.
	8.8 If you have stomach pain, nausea, vomiting, rapid breathing, or sweet, fruity-smelling breath, call your health care provider immediately or go to the emergency room.	Tell the patient ***If your blood glucose is low, eat a larger-than-usual bedtime snack.*** A change in insulin dose is needed if the finding is consistent.

continued on page 106

Document 7. Giant Diabetes Education Program Content Outline, continued

Concept	Information	Instructor's Notes
9. Benefits of monitoring	**9.1** Monitoring gives you information you need to make decisions as you care for your diabetes each day. Without this information, you are not able to make informed choices.	
	9.2 You can determine if you are hypoglycemic by testing your blood glucose. Sometimes you feel as if you are having a reaction, but you are not certain.	
	9.3 You can help detect and prevent nighttime hypoglycemic reactions by testing your blood glucose before bedtime. This is especially important if your blood glucose was lower than usual or you exercised more than usual that day.	Ask ***What are benefits of blood glucose monitoring for you?***
	9.4 You can determine the effects of a particular activity on your blood glucose by testing before and after the activity. For example, exercise, meals, taking medications.	Ask ***What do you need to be able to do with the results to make monitoring worthwhile for you?***
	9.5 Write down test results and bring to your appointments. Bring your meter also, so it can be downloaded.	Ask ***Is your blood glucose often high or low at a certain time of day?*** Put sample situations on a record form and ask questions about them.
	9.6 You need to decide personal benefits of monitoring.	All participants should have individual blood glucose parameters and know when to contact their health care teams. Remind participants to ask for these parameters.
	9.7 Monitoring alone will not control your blood glucose. You can learn to use the results of your tests to adjust your diet, medicine, and exercise.	
	9.8 Look for patterns in your blood glucose levels. Think about possible causes for your blood glucose patterns or changes from your usual pattern. This is the first step in using your results.	

continued on page 107

Document 7. Giant Diabetes Education Program Content Outline, continued

Concept	Information	Instructor's Notes
	9.9 Call your doctor or nurse if any problems arise between visits or if there are major changes in your results. Also call if you have low blood glucose for reasons you don't understand or if your blood glucose tests change suddenly and you don't know why or what to do.	
10. Goals of therapy	**10.1** Determine patient's target blood glucose levels based on physician's recommendations and patient characteristics. **10.2** Develop a monitoring plan for the patient.	
11. Selecting a meter if patient does not have one	**11.1** This selection should be based on the characteristics of the patient. **11.2** Instruct the patient on appropriate use of the meter. Demonstrate its use. **11.3** Demonstrate the use of the control solution and frequency of use.	

Source: Developed by Magaly Rodriguez de Bittner and used with permission from Giant Pharmacy.

Index

Note:
Italic *f* following a page number indicates a figure; italic *t* indicates a table.